Clinical Manual of Electroconvulsive Therapy

Mehul V. Mankad, M.D.

John L. Beyer, M.D.

Richard D. Weiner, M.D., Ph.D.

Andrew D. Krystal, M.D., M.S.

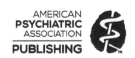

AMERICAN
PSYCHIATRIC
ASSOCIATION
PUBLISHING

If you would like to buy between 25 and 99 copies of this or any other APPI title, you are eligible for a 20% discount; please contact APPI Customer Service at appi@psych.org or 800-368-5777. If you wish to buy 100 or more copies of the same title, please e-mail us at bulksales@psych.org for a price quote.

Copyright © 2010 American Psychiatric Publishing, Inc.
ALL RIGHTS RESERVED

Manufactured in the United States of America on acid-free paper
24   23   22   21   20   5   4   3
First Edition

Typeset in Adobe's Garamond and Formata

American Psychiatric Publishing, Inc.
1000 Wilson Boulevard
Arlington, VA 22209-3901
www.appi.org

Library of Congress Cataloging-in-Publication Data
Clinical manual of electroconvulsive therapy / Mehul V. Mankad ... [et al.]. — 1st ed.
    p. ; cm.
    Includes bibliographical references and index.
    ISBN 978-1-58562-269-6 (alk. paper)
    1. Electroconvulsive therapy—Handbooks, manuals, etc. I. Mankad, Mehul V.
    [DNLM: 1. Electroconvulsive Therapy—instrumentation. 2. Electroconvulsive Therapy—methods. 3. Mental Disorders—therapy. 4. Seizures. WM 412 C6406 2010]
    RC485.C547 2010
    616.89′122—dc22
                                                                                    2009015496

British Library Cataloguing in Publication Data
A CIP record is available from the British Library.

Contents

List of Tables

List of Figures

About the Authors

John L. Beyer, M.D., is assistant professor of psychiatry and behavioral sciences at Duke University Medical Center in Durham, North Carolina.

Andrew D. Krystal, M.D., M.S., is professor of psychiatry and behavioral sciences at Duke University Medical Center in Durham, North Carolina.

Mehul V. Mankad, M.D., is clinical associate in psychiatry and behavioral sciences at Duke University Medical Center and staff psychiatrist at Durham Veterans Affairs Medical Center in Durham, North Carolina.

Richard D. Weiner, M.D., Ph.D., is professor of psychiatry and behavioral sciences at Duke University Medical Center and chief of the Mental Health Service Line at Durham Veterans Affairs Medical Center in Durham, North Carolina.

Disclosure of Competing Interests

The following contributors to this book have indicated a financial interest in or other affiliation with a commercial supporter, a manufacturer of a commercial product, a provider of a commercial service, a nongovernmental organization, and/or a government agency, as listed below:

John L. Beyer, M.D.—*Research support:* Eisai Pharmaceuticals, Elan Pharmaceuticals, Eli Lilly, Forest, Novartis, Sanofi-Synthelabo, Sonexa; *Advisory board:* Eli Lilly; *Speaker's bureau:* Schering-Plough (recently acquired by Merck)

Andrew D. Krystal, M.D., M.S.—*Grants/research support:* Astellas, Cephalon, Evotec, GlaxoSmithKline, Merck, National Institutes of Health, Neurocrine, Neuronetics, Pfizer, Respironics, Sepracor, Somaxon, Takeda, Transcept; *Consultant:* Actelion, Arena, Astellas, AstraZeneca, Axiom, Bristol-Myers Squibb, Cephalon, Eli Lilly, GlaxoSmithKline, Jazz, Johnson &

Johnson, King, Kingsdown, Merck, Neurocrine, Neurogen, Novartis, Organon, Ortho-McNeil-Janssen, Pfizer, Research Triangle Institute, Respironics, Roche, Sanofi-Aventis, Sepracor, Somaxon, Takeda, Transcept

Richard D. Weiner, M.D., Ph.D.—The author is co-inventor on a Duke patent licensed to MECTA Corp. He does not receive royalties for this.

Preface

Few treatments in psychiatry have experienced the longevity and unheralded effectiveness of electroconvulsive therapy (ECT). ECT remains the definitive treatment for a variety of mental disorders for a good reason: it is often effective when other treatments fail. At times, the effects of ECT can be lifesaving in their magnitude and rapid onset of action. However, in spite of the proven efficacy and safety of this standard treatment in psychiatry, its availability in individual communities is variable. Part of this disparity in access is related to misunderstanding by laypersons regarding the treatment and its potential adverse effects. Another limitation to access involves the inadequate number of psychiatrists who participate in ECT treatment programs. Adequate education and training of psychiatrists and their support staff are essential to ensure access to this vital treatment tool. In this capacity, we hope that the *Clinical Manual of Electroconvulsive Therapy* will help psychiatrists incorporate ECT into their clinical practice.

In 1985, *Electroconvulsive Therapy: A Programmed Text*, by Mark D. Glenn and Richard D. Weiner, was published. A second edition, by John L. Beyer, Richard D. Weiner, and Mark D. Glenn, followed in 1998. The intent of these texts was to provide the reader with a scheduled approach to understanding fundamental concepts underpinning ECT while providing practical, reproducible information to establish and maintain an ECT program. Since the publication of that second edition, another decade of ECT research and practice has passed. Ultra-brief pulse ECT, alternatives to established anesthesia regimens, and new ECT devices are some of the changes that have emerged. We are excited to incorporate the essence of the previous books into the *Clinical Manual of Electroconvulsive Therapy* while including discussion of important changes in the field.

In this text, we discuss several ECT devices and prescription medications. We are not recommending a specific device over another but firmly believe that the information provided helps potential ECT clinicians make informed choices regarding management of their ECT program resources. Also, no textbook can replace the careful, nuanced experience of learning a medical procedure under the supervision of a seasoned colleague. This volume is not meant to replace that indispensable aspect of medical education.

Acknowledgment

This endeavor could not have been possible without the support of our families, and we happily remain in their debt.

PART 1

Background

History of
Electroconvulsive Therapy

John L. Beyer, M.D.

Older Somatic Therapies

Until the 1930s, options for treatment of psychiatric patients were limited. Psychotherapy (primarily psychoanalysis) was the principal treatment for outpatients, but little more than custodial care or prevention of harm could be done for the more severe cases, which required inpatient management. Efforts to find useful somatic therapies ranged widely, but most of these therapies were ineffective. Hydrotherapy with cold packs, water therapy (continuous tub baths), prolonged sleep therapy, insulin coma, and Scotch douches were all attempts to use available means to treat patients (Endler and Persad 1988; Lebensohn 1999; Shorter and Healy 2007). Sedatives—primarily barbiturates, bromides, paraldehyde, and chloral hydrate—were the only medications available until the advent of antipsychotics and antidepressants in the 1950s. Overall, there was an attitude of general distrust from the public at large toward somatic therapies.

Chemical Convulsive Therapy

In 1934, Ladislas Joseph von Meduna, a Hungarian neuropsychiatrist, conducted the first experiments in treating patients with schizophrenia by inducing repeated seizures. Observational reports had circulated noting that symptoms of dementia praecox (schizophrenia) were diminished when patients developed epilepsy (e.g., after head traumas or neurological illnesses) and that patients with epilepsy had a low incidence of psychosis. Further, Meduna's own neuropathology studies found that the glial cell concentrations in the brains of patients with epilepsy were much higher than normal, whereas glial cell concentrations in the brains of patients with schizophrenia were much lower. Meduna hypothesized, therefore, that seizures may be "protective" against psychosis and that inducing convulsions in patients with schizophrenia could reduce their symptoms (Fink 2004). The idea that the induction of one illness could treat another was based on the accepted theory of biological antagonism (Fink 2001). A common example of successful biological antagonism treatment was the practice of inducing malarial fevers as a cure for patients with neurosyphilis. This procedure, introduced in 1917 by Professor Julius Wagner-Juaregg of Vienna, marked a major advance in medicine and was recognized as such when he was awarded the Nobel Prize for Medicine in 1928.

Interestingly, the observational reports of decreased psychosis in patients with epilepsy were incorrect. Research has shown that individuals with epilepsy are more likely than those without to have psychosis. Meduna apparently was aware of this, emphasizing not the chronic medical conditions (epilepsy and schizophrenia) as being antagonistic but rather the specific events of seizure-antagonizing psychotic symptoms (Fink 2004). Despite the questionable data and methodological theory, Meduna's early clinical trials were successful. They demonstrated a significant decrease in psychotic symptoms in patients treated with a series of induced seizures (with dramatic improvement especially noted in patients who appeared to have catatonia) (Fink 1984). The practice of convulsive therapy quickly spread throughout Europe and the United States (Shorter and Healy 2007).

Origins of Electroconvulsive Therapy

Initially, Meduna used pharmacological methods to induce seizure activity. He began with intramuscular injections of camphor, which was known to be a stimulant at lower doses. However, since camphor was painful and variable in its effect, he switched agents to pentylenetetrazol (Metrazol), a more refined synthetic substance. Although this method was effective in promoting seizures, it was still variable in its effects and had numerous side effects (especially a sense of panic). In 1937, the Italian neuropsychiatrists Ugo Cerletti and Lucio Bini began to induce seizures experimentally with electricity (Accornero 1988; Bini 1995; Shorter and Healy 2007). They found that seizures could be more easily induced and regulated with electricity than with pharmacological agents, thereby decreasing the number of missed or recurrent seizures. Electroconvulsive therapy (ECT) quickly replaced pentylenetetrazol as the method of inducing convulsions, and within a few years, ECT became the dominant somatic treatment not only for schizophrenia but also for major mood disorders (see Chapter 2, "Indications for Use").

Initially, the concept that grand mal seizures could be beneficial was considered dubious. Explanations for the effectiveness of ECT included the possibility that any benefit from the procedure was due to the "psychological" effect brought on by the dramatic and impressive efforts used to help the individual. This theory was tested in trials using sham ECT, in which the patients went through the full procedure for ECT but did not receive the stimulation or received only a subconvulsive dose. The U.K. Medical Research Council (Palmer 1981), the U.K. ECT Review Group (2003), and authors of a more recent Cochrane review (Tharyan and Adams 2005) reported that in randomized controlled trials of sham ECT compared with actual ECT, sham ECT was ineffective.

The focus again returned to the role of seizures for therapeutic efficacy. Meduna concluded that the manner in which a seizure was induced—via medication or electrical stimulation—did not matter as long as a full seizure was induced (Fink 2004). Ottosson (1960) found that when the intensity or duration of the seizures was varied, the seizures that were poorly organized or incomplete were less effective. Such studies supported the conclusion that anything that interfered with the grand mal seizure also interfered with the efficacy of the treatment. However, the mechanism of action behind this effect has still not been fully determined.

Patterns of Use

In the mid-1950s, the use of ECT began to decline and continued to do so for many years (Babigian and Guttmacher 1984; Shorter and Healy 2007). Two trends appear to have influenced this change. First, pharmacological antipsychotic, antidepressant, and (later) antimanic agents for the treatment of mental disorders were discovered and heralded as less intrusive alternatives to ECT. Second, ECT became the subject of a number of highly negative portrayals in the media (Jenkusky 1992). A negative image of ECT was sensationalized in the movie *One Flew Over the Cuckoo's Nest*, which demonstrated the use of unmodified ECT as a method of behavior control. Many other media presentations also represented ECT as a cruel and inhumane treatment in which attendants held an unwilling patient down while electricity was applied to the head, causing a dramatic and terrifying grand mal convulsion (see McDonald and Walter 2001 for a more in-depth discussion of ECT in American movies from 1948 to 1998). These images invoked fears of authoritarianism and social control during a time of social change in the United States that emphasized autonomy and distrust of the establishment. Such presentations also invoked fears of indiscriminate punishment by the inherent association with the electric chair. Unfortunately, many Americans still have this stigmatized view of ECT and its technique of administration, although recent media depictions have tended to be more realistic, positive, and supportive.

Increasingly, ECT is being recognized as a proven, effective, and even lifesaving intervention for patients with certain mental disorders when other treatments have had little or no effect. Furthermore, the technique of administering ECT now bears little resemblance to that used in the early days of treatment. Major innovations include the use of anesthesia, oxygenation, muscle relaxation, seizure monitoring, and other modifications discussed throughout this book. These innovations, based on extensive research over the past 70 years, have also served to make this very effective treatment much safer and more acceptable to patients who receive it (Lisanby 2007). These changes also have paved the way for the development of newer, nonpharmacological somatic therapies, such as vagal nerve stimulation and transcranial magnetic stimulation.

Evidence indicates that the decline in use of ECT has leveled off since the mid-1980s and that ECT use may be experiencing a modest resurgence (Munk-Olsen et al. 2006; Thompson et al. 1994). This phenomenon appears to be due to several factors. First, the innovations in ECT technique mentioned earlier have contributed to a growing acceptance of this modality by practitioners and patients alike (Dukakis and Tye 2006). Second, practitioners are increasingly realizing that despite the great promise of psychotropic medications, some patients with mental illnesses are intolerant to available drugs or have symptoms that are drug refractory. Finally, the speed of action of ECT compared with alternative treatments has become of increasing interest in the present era of managed care and ever-decreasing lengths of stay, at least for those patients whose illness is severe enough to require hospitalization. Abrams (2002) estimated that over 100,000 people receive ECT treatments in the United States each year.

References

Abrams R: Electroconvulsive Therapy, 4th Edition. New York, Oxford University Press, 2002

Accornero F: An eyewitness account of the discovery of electroshock. Convuls Ther 4:40–49, 1988

Babigian HM, Guttmacher LB: Epidemiologic considerations in electroconvulsive therapy. Arch Gen Psychiatry 41:246–253, 1984

Bini L: Professor Bini's notes on the first electro-shock experiment. Convuls Ther 11:260–261, 1995

Dukakis K, Tye L: The Healing Power of Electroconvulsive Therapy. New York, Penguin, 2006

Endler NS, Persad E: Electroconvulsive therapy: the myths and the realities. Toronto, ON, Hans Huber, 1988

Fink M: Meduna and the origins of convulsive therapy. Am J Psychiatry 141:1034–1041, 1984

Fink M: Convulsive therapy: a review of the first 55 years. J Affect Disord 63:1–15, 2001

Fink M: Induced seizures as psychiatric therapy: Ladislas Meduna's contribution in modern neuroscience. J ECT 20:133–136, 2004

Jenkusky SM: Public perception of electroconvulsive therapy: a historical review. Jefferson Journal of Psychiatry 10:2–11, 1992

Lebensohn ZM: The history of electroconvulsive therapy in the United States and its place in American psychiatry: a personal memoir. Compr Psychiatry 40:173–181, 1999

Lisanby SH: Electroconvulsive therapy for depression. N Engl J Med 357:1939–1945, 2007

McDonald A, Walter G: The portrayal of ECT in American movies. J ECT 17:264–274, 2001

Munk-Olsen T, Laursen TM, Videbech P, et al: Electroconvulsive therapy: predictors and trends in utilization from 1976 to 2000. J ECT 22:127–132, 2006

Ottosson JO: Experimental studies of the mode of action of electroconvulsive therapy. Acta Psychiatr Scand 35(suppl):1–141, 1960

Palmer RL: Electroconvulsive Therapy: An Appraisal. Oxford, UK, Oxford University Press, 1981

Shorter R, Healy D: Shock Therapy: A History of Electroconvulsive Treatment in Mental Illness. New Brunswick, NJ, Rutgers University Press, 2007

Tharyan P, Adams CE: Electroconvulsive therapy for schizophrenia. Cochrane Database of Systematic Reviews, Issue 2. Art. No.: CD000076. DOI: 10.1002/14651858. CD000076.pub2, 2005

Thompson JW, Weiner RD, Myers CP: Use of ECT in the United States in 1975, 1980, and 1986. Am J Psychiatry 151:1657–1661, 1994

The U.K. ECT Review Group: Efficacy and safety of electroconvulsive therapy in depressive disorders: a systematic review and meta-analysis. Lancet 361:799–808, 2003

2

Indications for Use

John L. Beyer, M.D.

ECT was initially developed for the treatment of patients with schizophrenia, but its success encouraged trials in patients with other psychiatric diseases. Not all trials were successful. In fact, the application of ECT in patients seeking treatment for homosexuality, drug addiction, alcoholism, phobias, and conversion reactions led to complaints that ECT practitioners were abusing patients, thus contributing to the stigma of ECT. However, as a result of the trial-and-error process, as well as subsequent scientific clinical studies, the use of ECT is now more systematized. Two major factors are now recognized in the decision to use ECT: 1) the diagnostic indications for which ECT is effective and 2) the timing of ECT use in the course of these disorders.

Diagnostic Indications

Mood Disorders

Major Depressive Disorder

Major depressive episodes are a severe epidemiological problem. Approximately 10%–15% of the U.S. population may suffer from this condition at some time during their lives. Patients with major depressive episodes experience profound alterations in sleep pattern, appetite, libido, body weight, and activity level, as well as mood (American Psychiatric Association 2000a). This diagnosis does not necessarily imply the absence of an initial precipitant to the present episode or an absence of concurrent mental disorders. However, the diagnosis of major depressive episodes does indicate that the depressive symptoms are severe, pervasive, and inappropriately prolonged (see Table 2–1).

By the 1940s, ECT had been found to be an extremely effective treatment for depression. When the first antidepressant medications were introduced in the 1950s, comparison studies suggested that ECT and antidepressants were comparable in efficacy. The ease of use of the medications (especially the newer antidepressant agents) led to the decline of ECT, or at least its lower hierarchical place in treatment algorithms.

Reexamination of the evidence has suggested that ECT may actually demonstrate a much more powerful antidepressant response than medications. Fink (2001) retrospectively reviewed the comparison studies and noted that significant type II statistical errors occurred because of the small sample sizes. He also argued that the possible increased efficacy of ECT may have face validity because of the fact that ECT is frequently efficacious when medications have failed, it is often used for the more severe forms of depression, and it has a much quicker speed of response.

Despite the proliferation of pharmacotherapy, successful treatment of major depressive episodes has been estimated at only 60%–70% (American Psychiatric Association 2000b). Clinical trials and comparative studies have shown ECT to be effective in all types of major depressive episodes. For primary major depressive episodes, the remission rate has been estimated at 80%–90% (American Psychiatric Association 2000b). Because of the strong antidepressant response observed in very ill patients, ECT was initially believed to be most effective in melancholic depression, a subtype of major depressive episodes that is associated with prominent vegetative symptoms (e.g., anhedonia, anorexia, psychomotor retardation, and worsened symptoms in the mornings). Some researchers have suggested that the degree of improvement with ECT is directly correlated with the severity of the depressive illness. Unfortunately, attempts to predict clinical response based on clinical symptoms, patient history, demographics, or other factors have been largely unsuccessful (Weiner and Coffey 1988). Evidence has suggested, how-

Table 2–1.   DSM-IV-TR criteria for major depressive episode

A. Five (or more) of the following symptoms have been present during the same 2-week period and represent a change from previous functioning; at least one of the symptoms is either (1) depressed mood or (2) loss of interest or pleasure.

Note: Do not include symptoms that are clearly due to a general medical condition, or mood-incongruent delusions or hallucinations.

(1) depressed mood most of the day, nearly every day, as indicated by either subjective report (e.g., feels sad or empty) or observation made by others (e.g., appears tearful).   Note: In children and adolescents, can be irritable mood.

(2) markedly diminished interest or pleasure in all, or almost all, activities most of the day, nearly every day (as indicated by either subjective account or observation made by others)

(3) significant weight loss when not dieting or weight gain (e.g., a change of more than 5% of body weight in a month), or decrease or increase in appetite nearly every day.   Note: In children, consider failure to make expected weight gains.

(4) insomnia or hypersomnia nearly every day

(5) psychomotor agitation or retardation nearly every day (observable by others, not merely subjective feelings of restlessness or being slowed down)

(6) fatigue or loss of energy nearly every day

(7) feelings of worthlessness or excessive or inappropriate guilt (which may be delusional) nearly every day (not merely self-reproach or guilt about being sick)

(8) diminished ability to think or concentrate, or indecisiveness, nearly every day (either by subjective account or as observed by others)

(9) recurrent thoughts of death (not just fear of dying), recurrent suicidal ideation without a specific plan, or a suicide attempt or a specific plan for committing suicide

B. The symptoms do not meet criteria for a mixed episode.

C. The symptoms cause clinically significant distress or impairment in social, occupational, or other important areas of functioning.

D. The symptoms are not due to the direct physiological effects of a substance (e.g., a drug of abuse, a medication) or a general medical condition (e.g., hypothyroidism).

E. The symptoms are not better accounted for by bereavement, i.e., after the loss of a loved one, the symptoms persist for longer than 2 months or are characterized by marked functional impairment, morbid preoccupation with worthlessness, suicidal ideation, psychotic symptoms, or psychomotor retardation.

Source.   Reprinted from American Psychiatric Association: *Diagnostic and Statistical Manual of Mental Disorders,* 4th Edition, Text Revision. Washington, DC, American Psychiatric Association, 2000. Copyright 2000, American Psychiatric Association. Used with permission.

ever, that the likelihood of response to ECT is diminished for patients whose depressive episodes occur in the context of a concurrent mental or medical disease (e.g., those with secondary depression) or who have been refractory to previous medication trials during the present episode of illness (Sackeim et al. 1990). Dombrovski et al. (2005) evaluated predictors of remission in depressed patients presenting for ECT treatment from 1993 to 1999. They found (unsurprisingly) that chronic depression/dysthymia and medication resistance were predictors for nonremission. Two indications that may predict a more powerful response are presence of acute catatonic features (see the section "Schizophrenia" later in this chapter) or delusions (Parker et al. 1992).

In 1975, Glassman et al. reported on the differential responses to imipramine of depressed patients with or without delusions. With imipramine treatment, only 3 of 13 patients with delusional depression responded, whereas 14 of 21 patients with nondelusional depression responded. Interestingly, 9 of the 10 unimproved patients with delusional depression recovered with subsequent ECT. Similar findings were reported by Avery and Lubrano (1979), who reevaluated the treatment responses of 437 patients with depression. Initially, all patients were given therapeutic doses of imipramine, and 247 (57%) recovered. The 190 patients who did not recover were then treated with bilateral ECT. Of these, 156 (72%) recovered. Subsequent evaluation found that among the patients with delusional depression, 83% improved with ECT compared with 40% with imipramine. When response was evaluated by depression severity, ECT response rate was 83% compared with 35% for the imipramine group among those patients with severe depression. Kroessler et al. (1985) evaluated the treatment responses of 597 patients with delusional depression from 17 studies. They found that the patients' response rate to tricyclic antidepressants alone was 34%, to antipsychotics alone was 51%, to combination tricyclic antidepressants-antipsychotics was 77%, and to ECT was 82%. It should also be noted that the efficacy of ECT in patients with highly treatment-resistant conditions, particularly those with comorbid mental illness, appears to be significantly less than reported in the context of research studies with rigorous entry criteria (Prudic et al. 2004). This phenomenon is important in terms of consent for ECT, given that many patients clinically referred for ECT may fall into such a category.

In the United States, 80%–90% of all ECT treatments are performed for the treatment of major depressive episodes. In a study reviewing use of ECT in Denmark from 1976 to 2000, the primary diagnosis for patients treated with ECT was also unipolar depression. However, patients with unipolar depression were only 65% of the total sample (Munk-Olsen et al. 2006). The authors noted that the trend in ECT use in Denmark over the past 25 years has been for an overall increased percentage of patients with unipolar depression relative to other diagnostic indications.

Table 2–2.   DSM-IV-TR criteria for manic episode

A.   A distinct period of abnormally and persistently elevated, expansive, or irritable mood, lasting at least 1 week (or any duration if hospitalization is necessary).

B.   During the period of mood disturbance, three (or more) of the following symptoms have persisted (four if the mood is only irritable) and have been present to a significant degree:

    (1)   inflated self-esteem or grandiosity

    (2)   decreased need for sleep (e.g., feels rested after only 3 hours of sleep)

    (3)   more talkative than usual or pressure to keep talking

    (4)   flight of ideas or subjective experience that thoughts are racing

    (5)   distractibility (i.e., attention too easily drawn to unimportant or irrelevant external stimuli)

    (6)   increase in goal-directed activity (either socially, at work or school, or sexually) or psychomotor agitation

    (7)   excessive involvement in pleasurable activities that have a high potential for painful consequences (e.g., engaging in unrestrained buying sprees, sexual indiscretions, or foolish business investments)

C.   The symptoms do not meet criteria for a mixed episode.

D.   The mood disturbance is sufficiently severe to cause marked impairment in occupational functioning or in usual social activities or relationships with others, or to necessitate hospitalization to prevent harm to self or others, or there are psychotic features.

E.   The symptoms are not due to the direct physiological effects of a substance (e.g., a drug of abuse, a medication, or other treatment) or a general medical condition (e.g., hyperthyroidism).

Note.   Manic-like episodes that are clearly caused by somatic antidepressant treatment (e.g., medication, electroconvulsive therapy, light therapy) should not count toward a diagnosis of bipolar I disorder.

Source.   Reprinted from American Psychiatric Association: *Diagnostic and Statistical Manual of Mental Disorders,* 4th Edition, Text Revision. Washington, DC, American Psychiatric Association, 2000. Copyright 2000, American Psychiatric Association. Used with permission.

Mania

In bipolar disorder, the "pole" opposite depression is mania. During a manic episode, a person's mood and energy are generally elevated such that his or her functioning and organization are impaired (American Psychiatric Association 2000a) (see Table 2–2). ECT is an effective treatment for acute mania. Reviews have reported improvement in approximately 80% of manic patients treated with ECT (Mukherjee et al. 1994). This finding is even more impressive considering that many of these patients were pharmacologically unresponsive.

When ECT was first introduced for the treatment of mania, the high mortality rates from exhaustion and from suicide were abruptly reduced, making ECT the primary treatment of the illness (Fink 2006; Ziskind et al. 1945). However, the widespread and successful use of lithium and other antimanic agents, often in combination with antipsychotic medications, has generally relegated ECT to use only in patients who are intolerant of or refractory to medications. This situation may represent an underutilization of ECT for patients with mania. Although early anecdotal evidence suggested that mania was more resistant to ECT or required more frequent treatments than depression, recent research suggests that this is untrue. Less research support is available for use of ECT in patients with mania than in those with depression or schizophrenia, but recent reports suggest that ECT should be considered in mania cases that are acutely treatment refractory (Sienaert and Peuskens 2006) or require aggressive therapy for maintenance stabilization (Nascimento et al. 2006). Furthermore, ECT may play a more significant role in the treatment of patients with delirious mania or in rapid-cycling manic states (Fink 2000).

Thought Disorders

Schizophrenia

Approximately 1% of the U. S. population has schizophrenia. This condition causes a progressive deterioration of the patient's ability to organize thoughts and to discriminate between reality and false perceptions (American Psychiatric Association 2000a) (see Table 2–3).

Although ECT was originally developed for the treatment of psychoses, physicians quickly realized that it was much more effective in treating mood dis-

Table 2–3. DSM-IV-TR diagnostic criteria for schizophrenia

A. *Characteristic symptoms:* Two (or more) of the following, each present for a significant portion of time during a 1-month period (or less if successfully treated):

(1) delusions

(2) hallucinations

(3) disorganized speech (e.g., frequent derailment or incoherence)

(4) grossly disorganized or catatonic behavior

(5) negative symptoms, i.e., affective flattening, alogia, or avolition

Note: Only one criterion A symptom is required if delusions are bizarre or hallucinations consist of a voice keeping up a running commentary on the person's behavior or thoughts, or two or more voices conversing with each other.

B. *Social/occupational dysfunction:* For a significant portion of the time since the onset of the disturbance, one or more major areas of functioning such as work, interpersonal relations, or self-care are markedly below the level achieved prior to the onset (or when the onset is in childhood or adolescence, failure to achieve expected level of interpersonal, academic, or occupational achievement).

C. *Duration:* Continuous signs of the disturbance persist for at least 6 months. This 6-month period must include at least 1 month of symptoms (or less if successfully treated) that meet criterion A (i.e., active-phase symptoms) and may include periods of prodromal or residual symptoms. During these prodromal or residual periods, the signs of the disturbance may be manifested by only negative symptoms or two or more symptoms listed in criterion A present in an attenuated form (e.g., odd beliefs, unusual perceptual experiences).

D. *Schizoaffective and mood disorder exclusion:* Schizoaffective disorder and mood disorder with psychotic features have been ruled out because either (1) no major depressive, manic, or mixed episodes have occurred concurrently with the active-phase symptoms; or (2) if mood episodes have occurred during active-phase symptoms, their total duration has been brief relative to the duration of the active and residual periods.

E. *Substance/general medical condition exclusion:* The disturbance is not due to the direct physiological effects of a substance (e.g., a drug of abuse, a medication) or a general medical condition.

F. *Relationship to a pervasive developmental disorder:* If there is a history of autistic disorder or another pervasive developmental disorder, the additional diagnosis of schizophrenia is made only if prominent delusions or hallucinations are also present for at least a month (or less if successfully treated).

Table 2–3.   DSM-IV-TR diagnostic criteria for schizophrenia

Classification of longitudinal course (can be applied only after at least 1 year has elapsed since the initial onset of active-phase symptoms):

Episodic with interepisode residual symptoms (episodes are defined by the reemergence of prominent psychotic symptoms); *also specify if:* with prominent negative symptoms

Episodic with no interepisode residual symptoms

Continuous (prominent psychotic symptoms are present throughout the period of observation); *also specify if:* with prominent negative symptoms

Single episode in partial remission; *also specify if:* with prominent negative symptoms

Single episode in full remission

Other or unspecified pattern

Source.   Reprinted from American Psychiatric Association: *Diagnostic and Statistical Manual of Mental Disorders,* 4th Edition, Text Revision. Washington, DC, American Psychiatric Association, 2000. Copyright 2000, American Psychiatric Association. Used with permission.

orders than schizophrenia. In fact, a review of early cases suggests that the remarkable treatment response seen may have been in patients with catatonia (a subtype of schizophrenia in which the person becomes mute and stuporous, often adopting bizarre postures, or demonstrates excessive activity). This condition is now frequently associated with mood disorders (Abrams and Taylor 1976).

With the development of effective antipsychotic agents in the 1950s, resulting clinical trials found that ECT alone is significantly less effective than antipsychotic medication for patients with schizophrenia, at least as a first-line treatment (Krueger and Sackeim 1995; Small 1985; Tharyan and Adams 2005). In acutely ill patients with nonchronic schizophrenia, the estimated rate of remission for those treated with ECT ranges between 40% and 80% (Small 1985; Weiner and Coffey 1988), with a more likely response in patients who exhibit catatonia or prominent affective symptoms (König and Glatter-Götz 1990). In a study of first-episode schizophrenia comparing ECT and antipsychotic treatment groups, catatonic patients who were not medication responsive and violent patients were treated with ECT (Uçok and Cakr 2006). Although patients in the ECT group had a higher Brief Psychiatric Rating Scale score at admission, they ended up having a lower score at discharge. Unfortunately, the 1-year follow-up found that relapses were frequent.

Patients with chronic schizophrenia have a much lower rate of remission or significant improvement (only 5%–10%), and in the United States only

5%–10% of all ECT courses are now administered to patients with this disorder. However, in many parts of the developing world where ECT is available and inexpensive, schizophrenia continues to be a more frequent clinical indication for the use of ECT than in the United States (Agarwal et al. 1992).

A lack of consensus currently exists on when to use ECT in the treatment of individuals with schizophrenia. The American Psychiatric Association's Committee on Electroconvulsive Therapy recommended the use of ECT in patients who have a history of a favorable response to ECT or who have abrupt psychotic exacerbations, catatonic schizophrenia, or schizoaffective disorder (where there is a mixture of schizophrenia and mood disorder symptoms); however, the committee recommends against ECT if "negative" symptoms of schizophrenia (e.g., withdrawal, mutism, poor self-care, flat affect) predominate (American Psychiatric Association 2001). In its second report, the Royal College of Psychiatrists' Special Committee on ECT also recommended ECT for patients with schizophrenia who have positive, affective, or catatonic symptoms (Royal College of Psychiatrists 1995). In contrast, the National Institute for Clinical Excellence (2003) in the United Kingdom does not recommend the general use of ECT for people with schizophrenia, although catatonia is considered an indication.

Recently, interest has been growing in the use of ECT as part of a combination treatment. Convincing evidence indicates that concurrent antipsychotic medication and ECT may be more effective than either treatment alone (Klapheke 1993; Krueger and Sackeim 1995; Sajatovic and Meltzer 1993; Weiner and Coffey 1988). In a meta-analysis of studies evaluating the efficacy of combined ECT and antipsychotic therapy in schizophrenia, Painuly and Chakrabarti (2006) found that the combination might be better than antipsychotic drugs used alone in the first few weeks of treatment for schizophrenia; the main benefit of adding ECT appeared to be an acceleration of treatment response. Braga and Petrides (2005) reviewed the literature and concluded that the combination is a safe and efficacious treatment strategy for patients with schizophrenia, especially those refractory to conventional treatments.

Chanpattana and Andrade (2006) have advocated the use of continuation ECT combined with maintenance antipsychotic medication as providing better treatment outcomes than either treatment alone (including improving the patient's quality of life and functioning in the long term). In one well-conducted study, Chanpattana et al. (1999) found that combination therapy using ECT and antipsychotics was extremely effective in preventing relapse (number needed to treat=2; 95% confidence interval=1.5–2.5). This finding is remarkable considering that 1) the comparison was not with placebo, but rather against active treatments, and 2) the subjects were treatment resistant to antipsychotics. The potency of this combination therapy has caused some (e.g., Hertzman 1992) to call for a reconsideration of ECT on even a primary basis in patients with schizophrenia. Some particularly impressive results have been obtained with clozapine nonresponders who then received the combination of ECT and clozapine (Kho et al. 2004).

Schizoaffective Disorder

Given the mood component inherent in schizoaffective disorder, the role for ECT in the treatment of this complex condition is clear. In those patients who do not respond adequately to psychopharmacology, ECT may serve an adjunctive role in the treatment of acute symptoms. The use of ECT in patients with schizoaffective disorder is particularly relevant in the context of acute mood symptoms (i.e., depressive or manic symptoms co-occurring with psychosis or in the absence of psychosis). Given the frequent use of mood stabilizer medications from the anticonvulsant class in patients with schizoaffective disorder, attention must be paid to the potentially higher seizure threshold that may be present. The risks and benefits of suspending mood stabilizers with anticonvulsant properties during an index course of ECT in patients with schizoaffective disorder is a clinical decision that varies across individual cases.

Other Psychiatric Disorders

Because of its success in treating the major mood disorders and acute schizophrenia, ECT has been tried in patients with a variety of other mental disorders. No compelling evidence supports the effectiveness of ECT in the treatment of dysthymia, anxiety disorders, substance abuse disorders, eating disorders, or personality disorders (Weiner and Coffey 1988); however, the practitioner should always bear in mind that a diagnostic indication for ECT may coexist with these and other psychiatric conditions. Interestingly, in media portrayals of ECT, the most common reason for ECT administration is to "treat" antisocial behavior, a diagnosis for which ECT has long been known as ineffective. McDonald and Walter (2001) found that major depression, the most frequently prescribed indication for ECT, was the diagnostic criterion in only 3 of 20 movies that dealt with ECT.

General Medical Disorders

ECT has selective neurobiological effects that may help in the treatment of certain medical conditions, although a referral should be considered only for individuals who have been refractory to or intolerant of other therapies. Neuroleptic malignant syndrome (Bhanushali and Tuite 2004; Ghaziuddin et al. 2002; Ozer et al. 2005; Trollor and Sachdev 1999), refractory Parkinson's disease (Fregni et al. 2005; Ozer et al. 2005), some forms of intractable epilepsy (Lisanby et al. 2001), and certain endocrinopathies (hypopituitarism) (Pitts and Patterson 1979) have been documented to be responsive to ECT when other therapies have failed (Weiner and Coffey 1993). Parkinson's disease appears to respond especially well, particularly when the "on-off" syndrome is present (Faber and Trimble 1991). Unfortunately, relief from those symptoms may last only a few weeks to months, although a more prolonged effect may occur with the use of maintenance ECT (see Chapter 13, "Maintenance ECT").

Timing of ECT Use

Primary Versus Secondary Use of ECT

In general, ECT can be considered either a primary or a secondary treatment (American Psychiatric Association 2001). Primary use of ECT is usually considered in four types of situations: 1) when an urgent need (either psychiatrically or medically) for a rapid response exists, 2) when ECT poses less risk than other treatment alternatives, 3) when the patient has a history of better response to ECT than to other treatments, or 4) when the patient has a strong preference for its use. The majority of patients referred for ECT do not meet these criteria. ECT is conducted as a secondary treatment when 1) the patient has had a poor response or intolerance to alternative treatments or 2) the patient's clinical condition has deteriorated to the point that an urgent need for rapid response is present.

In recent years, efforts have been made to identify good clinical practice by creating treatment algorithms based on evidence-based medicine and expert opinion. ECT has been included in a number of the published algorithms for mood disorders (Beale and Kellner 2000), but it is recommended at different stages of treatment. Also, different algorithms may advise the use of ECT based on severity of illness, previous medication trials, identified symptoms of the mood disorder, or clinical experience.

ECT in Children and Adolescents

Because the use of ECT is rare in children and uncommon in adolescents, information on efficacy and adverse effects is extremely limited. However, available data suggest that diagnostic indications for the use of ECT in children and adolescents are the same as those for adults (Bertagnoli and Borchardt 1990). The limited use of ECT for treatment of mental disorders in children and adolescents is primarily due to four factors: 1) a general reluctance to use what are perceived to be drastic measures with children, 2) child psychiatrists' lack of experience with ECT, 3) a concern that inducing seizures may be "more toxic" in children (although data supporting this concern are not compelling), and 4) the existence of statutory regulations in some states that prevent or restrict the use of ECT in minors of certain ages. Because of these factors, most practitioners are reluctant to refer minors for ECT, particularly in the case of prepubertal children.

Because of the relative lack of data regarding the use of ECT in youth, the American Psychiatric Association (2001) recommends that prior to using ECT in an adolescent younger than age 18 years, a physician should seek a second opinion from a psychiatrist who is experienced in treating minors. Two such consultations are recommended for children younger than age 12 years. Guidelines for use of ECT in adolescents have been developed by the American Academy of Child and Adolescent Psychiatry (Ghaziuddin et al. 2004).

ECT in the Elderly

Since the early 1990s, the percentage of patients receiving ECT who are elderly appears to be increasing (Glen and Scott 1999; Thompson et al. 1994). This phenomenon is due in part to the overall increase in the number of older individuals in the general population, the severity of impairment that is associated with many mental disorders in elderly patients, and changing attitudes toward ECT (Consensus Development Conference 1993).

Some reports suggest that ECT is particularly effective in treating late-life depression (Flint and Rifat 1998). In a Cochrane review on the use of ECT in elderly patients with depression, Stek et al. (2003) reported that the randomized evidence on the efficacy and safety of ECT in this population is sparse. One trial concluded that actual ECT was superior to simulated ECT, but the study had several methodological problems and requires replication (O'Leary et al. 1994). In a review of the larger research literature (including nonrandomized studies), van der Wurff et al. (2003) found that the data more strongly supported the efficacy of ECT in depressed elderly patients than in younger patients. Unfortunately, the efficacy and safety of ECT in subpopulations of depressed elderly patients (subjects with comorbid dementia, Parkinson's disease, cerebrovascular disease) are not well known.

The use of ECT in elderly patients is generally safe, but it does present some challenges (Greenberg and Fink 1992; van der Wurff et al. 2003). The literature includes many reports of serious complications that may be related to ECT. These complications may be due to the fact that older patients have more medical illnesses, which may increase the risks of ECT. Patients with preexisting cerebral disease may have a greater likelihood of ECT-related cognitive losses. Medications used at the time of ECT treatment may require adjustment in accordance with alterations in the patient's pharmacokinetics. In addition, the seizure threshold is usually higher for elderly patients, often requiring a higher electrical stimulus intensity to produce an adequate seizure.

Remission Versus Cure

When reviewing indications for ECT, the clinician needs to understand that a course of ECT induces a remission of an episode of illness. It does not cure mental illness any more than antidepressant medications cure depression or antipsychotic agents cure psychosis. The risk of recurrence remains high; therefore, the practitioner must also address issues of post-ECT continuation treatment (see Chapter 13, "Maintenance ECT").

References

Abrams R, Taylor MA: Catatonia: a prospective clinical study. Arch Gen Psychiatry 33:579–581, 1976

Agarwal AK, Andrade C, Reddy MV: The practice of ECT in India: issues relating to the administration of ECT. Indian J Psychiatry 34:285–298, 1992

American Psychiatric Association: Diagnostic and Statistical Manual of Mental Disorders, 4th Edition, Text Revision. Washington, DC, American Psychiatric Association, 2000a

American Psychiatric Association: Practice guideline for the treatment of patients with major depressive disorder (revision). Am J Psychiatry 157:1–45, 2000b

American Psychiatric Association: The Practice of Electroconvulsive Therapy: Recommendations for Treatment, Training, and Privileging (A Task Force Report of the American Psychiatric Association), 2nd Edition. Washington, DC, American Psychiatric Publishing, 2001

Avery D, Lubrano A: Depression treated with imipramine and ECT: the DeCarolis study reconsidered. Am J Psychiatry 136:559–562, 1979

Beale MD, Kellner CH: ECT in the treatment algorithms: no need to save the best for last. J ECT 16:1–2, 2000

Bertagnoli MW, Borchardt CM: A review of ECT for children and adolescents. J Am Acad Child Adolesc Psychiatry 29:302–307, 1990

Bhanushali MJ, Tuite PJ: The evaluation and management of patients with neuroleptic malignant syndrome. Neurol Clin 22:389–411, 2004

Braga RJ, Petrides G: The combined use of electroconvulsive therapy and antipsychotics in patients with schizophrenia. J ECT 21:75–83, 2005

Chanpattana W, Andrade C: ECT for treatment-resistant schizophrenia: a response from the Far East to the UK. NICE report. J ECT 22:4–12, 2006

Chanpattana W, Chakrabhand ML, Sackeim HA, et al: Continuation ECT in treatment-resistant schizophrenia: a controlled study. J ECT 15:178–192, 1999

Consensus Development Conference: Diagnosis and treatment of depression in late life: the NIH Consensus Development Conference statement. Psychopharmacol Bull 29:87–100, 1993

Dombrovski AY, Mulsant BH, Haskett RF, et al: Predictors of remission after electroconvulsive therapy in unipolar major depression. J Clin Psychiatry 66:1043–1049, 2005

Faber R, Trimble MR: Electroconvulsive therapy in Parkinson's disease and other movement disorders. Mov Disord 6:293–303, 1991

Fink M: Electroshock revisited. Am Sci 88:162–167, 2000

Fink M: Convulsive therapy: a review of the first 55 years. J Affect Disord 63:1–15, 2001

Fink M: ECT in therapy-resistant mania: does it have a place? Bipolar Disord 8:307–309, 2006

Flint AJ, Rifat SL: The treatment of psychotic depression in later life: a comparison of pharmacotherapy and ECT. Int J Geriatr Psychiatry 13:23–28, 1998

Fregni F, Simon DK, Wu A, et al: Non-invasive brain stimulation for Parkinson's disease: a systematic review and meta-analysis of the literature. J Neurol Neurosurg Psychiatry 76:1614–1623, 2005

Ghaziuddin N, Alkhouri I, Champine D, et al: ECT treatment of malignant catatonia/NMS in an adolescent: a useful lesson in delayed diagnosis and treatment. J ECT 18:95–98, 2002

Ghaziuddin N, Kutcher SP, Knapp P, et al: Practice parameter for use of electroconvulsive therapy with adolescents. J Am Acad Child Adolesc Psychiatry 43:1521–1539, 2004

Glassman AH, Kantor SJ, Shostak M: Depression, delusions, and drug response. Am J Psychiatry 132:716–719, 1975

Glen T, Scott A: Rates of electroconvulsive therapy use in Edinburgh 1992–1997. J Affect Disord 54:81–85, 1999

Greenberg L, Fink M: The use of electroconvulsive therapy in geriatric patients. Clin Geriatr Med 8:349–354, 1992

Hertzman M: ECT and neuroleptics as primary treatment for schizophrenia (editorial). Biol Psychiatry 31:217–220, 1992

Kho KH, Blansjaar BA, de Vries S, et al: Electroconvulsive therapy for the treatment of clozapine nonresponders suffering from schizophrenia. Eur Arch Psychiatry Clin Neurosci 254:372–379, 2004

Klapheke MM: Combining ECT and antipsychotic agents: benefits and risks. Convuls Ther 9:241–255, 1993

König P, Glatter-Götz U: Combined electroconvulsive and neuroleptic therapy in schizophrenia refractory to neuroleptics. Schizophr Res 3:351–354, 1990

Kroessler D: Relative efficacy rates for therapies of delusional depression. Convuls Ther 1:173–182, 1985

Krueger RB, Sackeim HA: Electroconvulsive therapy and schizophrenia, in Schizophrenia. Edited by Hirsch SR, Weinberger DR. Cambridge, MA, Blackwell, 1995

Lisanby SH, Bazil CW, Resor SR, et al: ECT in the treatment of status epilepticus. J ECT 17:210–215, 2001

McDonald A, Walter G: The portrayal of ECT in American movies. J ECT 17:264–274, 2001

Mukherjee S, Sackeim HA, Schnur DB: Electroconvulsive therapy of acute manic episodes: a review of 50 years' experience. Am J Psychiatry 151:169–176, 1994

Munk-Olsen T, Laursen TM, Videbech P, et al: Electroconvulsive therapy: predictors and trends in utilization from 1976 to 2000. J ECT 22:127–132, 2006

Nascimento AL, Appolinario JC, Segenreich D, et al: Maintenance electroconvulsive therapy for recurrent refractory mania. Bipolar Disord 8:301–303, 2006

National Institute for Clinical Excellence: Guidance on the Use of Electroconvulsive Therapy: NICE Technology Appraisal Guidance 59. London: National Institute for Clinical Excellence, 2003

O'Leary DA, Gill D, Gregory S, et al: The effectiveness of real versus simulated electroconvulsive therapy in depressed elderly patients. Int J Geriatr Psychiatry 9:567–571, 1994

Ozer F, Meral H, Aydin B, et al: Electroconvulsive therapy in drug-induced psychiatric states and neuroleptic malignant syndrome. J ECT 21:125–127, 2005

Painuly N, Chakrabarti S: Combined use of electroconvulsive therapy and antipsychotics in schizophrenia: the Indian evidence. A review and a meta-analysis. J ECT 22:59–66, 2006

Parker G, Roy K, Hadzi-Pavlovic D, et al: Psychotic (delusional) depression: a meta-analysis of physical treatments. J Affect Disord 24:17–24, 1992

Pitts FN Jr, Patterson CW: Electroconvulsive therapy for iatrogenic hypothalamic-hypopituitarism (CRF-ACTH type). Am J Psychiatry 136:1074–1077, 1979

Prudic J, Olfson M, Marcus SC, et al: Effectiveness of electroconvulsive therapy in community settings. Biol Psychiatry 55:301–312, 2004

Royal College of Psychiatrists: The ECT Handbook: The Second Report of the Royal College of Psychiatrists' Special Committee on ECT. London: Royal College of Psychiatrists, 1995

Sackeim HA, Prudic J, Devanand DP, et al: The impact of medication resistance and continuation pharmacotherapy on relapse following response to electroconvulsive therapy in major depression. J Clin Psychopharmacol 10:96–104, 1990

Sajatovic M, Meltzer HY: The effect of short-term electroconvulsive treatment plus neuroleptics in treatment-resistant schizophrenia and schizoaffective disorder. Convuls Ther 9:167–175, 1993

Sienaert P, Peuskens J: Electroconvulsive therapy: an effective therapy of medication-resistant bipolar disorder. Bipolar Disord 8:304–306, 2006

Small JG: Efficacy of electroconvulsive therapy in schizophrenia, mania, and other disorders, I: schizophrenia. Convuls Ther 1:263–270, 1985

Stek M, van der Wurff FB, Hoogendijk W, et al: Electroconvulsive therapy (ECT) for the depressed elderly. Cochrane Database of Systematic Reviews, Issue 2. Art. No.: CD003593. DOI: 10.1002/14651858.CD003593, 2003

Tharyan P, Adams CE: Electroconvulsive therapy for schizophrenia. Cochrane Database of Systematic Reviews, Issue 2. Art. No.: CD000076. DOI: 10.1002/14651858.CD000076.pub2, 2005

Thompson JW, Weiner RD, Myers CP: Use of ECT in the United States in 1975, 1980, and 1986. Am J Psychiatry 151:1657–1661, 1994

Trollor JN, Sachdev PS: Electroconvulsive treatment of neuroleptic malignant syndrome: a review and report of cases. Aust N Z J Psychiatry 33:650–659, 1999

Uçok A, Cakr S: Electroconvulsive therapy in first-episode schizophrenia. J ECT 22:38–42, 2006

van der Wurff FB, Stek ML, Hoogendijk WJ, et al: The efficacy and safety of ECT in depressed older adults: a literature review. Int J Geriatr Psychiatry 18:894–904, 2003

Weiner RD, Coffey CE: Indications for use of electroconvulsive therapy, in Review of Psychiatry, Vol 7. Edited by Frances AJ, Hales RE. Washington, DC, American Psychiatric Press, 1988, pp 458–481

Weiner RD, Coffey CE: Electroconvulsive therapy in the medical and neurologic patient, in Psychiatric Care of the Medical Patient. Edited by Stoudemire A, Fogel BS. New York, Oxford University Press, 1993, pp 207–224

Ziskind E, Somerfeld-Ziskind E, Ziskind L: Metrazol and electric convulsive therapy of the affective psychoses: a controlled series of observations covering a period of five years. Arch Neurol Psychiatry 53:212–217, 1945

3

Patient Referral and Evaluation

John L. Beyer, M.D.

Mehul V. Mankad, M.D.

As discussed in previous chapters, ECT is a powerful treatment for mental illness. However, while it holds the promise of substantial benefit, ECT also has the potential for significant risk. Therefore, when considering ECT as part of the treatment plan for an identified patient, the physician needs to fully assess the risks and benefits of the procedure for that patient (American Psychiatric Association 2001; Klapheke 1997). This chapter reviews the process for making this assessment, focusing especially on information that must be obtained to conduct the risk-benefit analysis and identify the information that must be sought that will affect the selection of ECT practice.

Pre-ECT Evaluation and Consultation

Because contemporary ECT is a sophisticated medical procedure, all patients referred for this treatment must first be evaluated by a physician fully trained and privileged to administer ECT in the applicable facility (American Psychiatric Association 2001). This evaluation has five goals:

1. Obtain a complete psychiatric history and delineate the indication for ECT.
2. Review the patient's preexisting medical conditions and ongoing treatments, and determine what further evaluation, testing, or consultation is needed to evaluate potential risk levels.
3. Recommend appropriate modifications of the ECT procedure to minimize risks and maximize benefits.
4. Make a risk-benefit comparison of all viable treatment options.
5. Initiate the informed consent process.

Before proceeding with ECT treatment, the practitioner must first determine that the patient has an ECT-responsive condition and that the time to intervene with ECT is appropriate (see Chapter 2, "Indications for Use"). To perform this task, the practitioner will find a detailed history of the patient's present illness and previous psychiatric treatments to be extremely useful. If ECT has been used previously, information should be gathered on the details of that treatment, including electrical parameters, electrode placement, number of treatments, duration and/or quality of seizures, and medications used at the time of the treatments. This information will be useful in determining the optimum medication and stimulus dosing parameters at the time of the first treatment (see Chapter 5, "Clinical Applications," and Chapter 6, "Anesthetics and Other Medications").

Medical Assessment

A detailed medical history and physical examination are important to assess and minimize any potential risks that might be associated with ECT. A thorough psychiatric evaluation forms the basis of the history consultation. The history taking should include particular attention to the patient's handedness (which may guide electrode placement) and dentition; any history of head trauma, spontaneous seizures, or other neurological illnesses; and previous adverse reaction to general anesthesia, which is also relevant to preparation for ECT. Postoperative nausea and vomiting are relatively common sequelae of general anesthesia and can be addressed with medication prior to each treatment. Because of the nearly ubiquitous use of succinylcholine for muscle relaxation in ECT, a personal or family history of pseudocholinesterase deficiency or malignant hyperthermia should be communicated to the anesthesia team prior to the first scheduled treatment.

Table 3–1. Medical conditions that increase risk from ECT

- Recent intracranial hemorrhage
- Recent thromboembolic stroke
- Intracranial lesion (tumor or infection) causing mass effect
- Recent myocardial infarction, particularly if sequelae are present
- Unstable angina or decompensating heart failure
- Unstable vertebral fracture

Although no absolute contraindications to ECT have been determined, some medical conditions are known to increase the risk from the treatment (see Table 3–1). In general, the psychiatrist performing the ECT consultation should be aware of any history or symptoms indicating that the patient may have one of these conditions.

In addition, the physician performing the ECT procedure should conduct a physical examination with special focus on areas important for the procedure (Tess and Smetana 2009). The practitioner should examine the scalp for evidence of cranial defects or scalp disease (which may affect electrode placement) and should evaluate the patient's dentition. Loose or fragile teeth may require extraction, modification of the use of the bite block, or production of a protective oral prosthesis prior to initiation of ECT (McCall et al. 1992; Minneman 1995).

Significant medical problems, such as arrhythmias, severe hypertension, congestive heart failure, large aneurysms, or insulin-dependent diabetes mellitus, may require specialized medical consultation. Neurological consultation should be considered when problems related to head trauma, intracerebral tumor, stroke, epilepsy, or cerebrovascular malformations are uncovered. Also, because ECT has been associated with a transient increase in intraocular pressure (Edwards et al. 1990), an ophthalmology consultation is needed for the patient with closed-angle glaucoma, poorly controlled open-angle glaucoma, or retinal detachment.

When conferring with any specialized medical consultant, the referring physician must be specific about what information is desired. The consultant should not be asked to "medically clear" the patient for ECT, because only the patient's attending psychiatrist and ECT practitioner are in a position to make a full risk-benefit analysis. Instead, the consultant should be asked to assess

Table 3–2.   Required and suggested laboratory examinations

Required laboratory examinations	Suggested laboratory examinations where specifically indicated
Complete blood count	Thyroid-stimulating hormone test
Basic metabolic panel	Liver function tests
	Drug levels (lithium, valproic acid, carbamazepine)
	Prothrombin time/ Partial thromboplastin time/ International normalized ratio
	Electrocardiogram
	Chest X ray
	Neuroimaging (computed tomography or magnetic resonance imaging)
	Electroencephalogram
	Neuropsychological testing

the pertinent risks associated with the specific medical condition leading to the consultation and to make recommendations as to how such risks can be minimized.

Laboratory Tests and Special Examinations

The medical workup prior to ECT, as for any surgical or anesthetic procedure, should be consistent with the patient's history, symptoms, and age. Required laboratory tests vary with each patient, but a minimal screening battery should include hematocrit or hemoglobin, serum electrolytes, and electrocardiogram (American Psychiatric Association 2001) (see Table 3–2). Recently, however, the need for routine serum electrolytes and electrocardiograms in healthy young adults has been questioned. Several studies have analyzed Holter monitor recordings before and after ECT but have not found any significant effects in heart rate variability, frequency of ventricular or supraventricular events, or changes in ST segments due to ECT (Rasmussen et al. 2004; Takada et al. 2005; Troup et al. 1978). Overall, the literature has reported general cardiac safety with the use of ECT in subjects without cardiac disease. The treatment preparations for patients with a history of cardiac disease are discussed in the section on special medical conditions later in this chapter.

Table 3–3. Example of pre-ECT evaluation protocol

Procedure	Routine	Age > 40 years	Cardio-vascular disease	Pulmonary disease	Heavy smoking history
Psychiatric examination	X	X	X	X	X
ECT consult	X	X	X	X	X
Anesthesia evaluation	X	X	X	X	X
Informed consent	X	X	X	X	X
Hemoglobin/hematocrit	X	X	X	X	X
Serum electrolytes		X	X	X	
Electrocardiogram		X	X	X	X
Chest X ray			X	X	X

Because of the potential for memory impairment as a result of the ECT procedure, at least a bedside measure of cognitive function, including memory performance, should be administered prior to initiating ECT. At the time of this writing, only a small fraction of facilities utilize formal neuropsychological testing prior to ECT, although recommendations have been made for those who wish to do so (Porter et al. 2008). Few facilities also routinely require a laboratory assessment of cerebral integrity (e.g., electroencephalogram, head computed tomography, or brain magnetic resonance imaging) prior to the ECT procedure. However, such testing should always be considered for any patient who has evidence of a preexisting cerebral abnormality.

In the remote past, ECT practitioners recommended that all patients receive spinal X rays, but the introduction of muscle relaxants has negated the need for routine radiological procedures of this type. However, X rays should be considered if the patient has a history of musculoskeletal symptoms or disease involving the spine or adjacent structures.

Pre-ECT evaluation protocols, like the one shown in Table 3–3, have been implemented at many facilities to maintain quality medical care but decrease excess laboratory use. Appropriate tests, coupled with appropriate medical history and physical examination, will ensure that an adequate evaluation of the patient's medical status has been conducted.

Inpatient Versus Outpatient ECT

In general, ECT is a safe and effective treatment for patients in inpatient and outpatient settings. A number of factors should be kept in mind when considering the environment in which ECT is offered. At the clinical level, symptom severity may necessitate an inpatient hospitalization regardless of whether ECT is pursued. Acute suicidal ideation, uncontrolled psychotic delusions, or other severe psychiatric presentations may require that a patient be admitted to a psychiatric unit prior to initiation of ECT. Because the degree of symptom severity may be unclear prior to outpatient consultation for ECT, it is helpful to have a clear protocol identified for patients to be admitted from the outpatient ECT consultation area to an inpatient psychiatric unit as the need may arise. If the patient can be managed psychiatrically as an outpatient, ECT may be offered in the outpatient setting. In addition, some patients who begin ECT as inpatients may no longer require hospitalization for their primary psychiatric symptoms during their course of ECT. Those patients may be transferred to the outpatient ECT setting to complete their index course or to pursue maintenance ECT.

Referrals for ECT may arise for inpatients admitted to psychiatric units who were not specifically considered for ECT prior to admission. Educational material (pamphlets, informational video, etc.) can be made available to inpatient psychiatrists and nurses so they can initiate the discussion about ECT with patients prior to formal consultation. To facilitate this process, continuing medical education regarding ECT should be encouraged for inpatient health care providers who do not directly participate in the delivery of ECT.

Anesthesia Evaluation

Because general anesthesia and muscular relaxation are used during ECT, an anesthesia preoperative evaluation should be obtained. Any history of gastric reflux, personal or familial problems with anesthesia or surgery, and all current medications or allergies should be documented. A patient with pseudocholinesterase deficiency may have an impaired metabolism of the muscle relaxant succinylcholine during ECT, resulting in prolonged apnea. A test for pseudocholinesterase activity may be required if the patient has a personal or family history of prolonged apnea when exposed to generalized anesthesia. Barbiturate anesthesia may pose a problem for patients with porphyria. The

American Society of Anesthesiologists has graded various medical conditions related to anesthetic risk; special care should be taken in any patient who may be evaluated as class 4 or 5. For potentially high-risk patients, the anesthesia consultant should see the patient 1 or 2 days in advance because further testing or consultations may be indicated, and treatment modifications or special preparations may be needed prior to the treatment. Anesthesia with respect to the ECT procedure is discussed in greater detail in Chapter 6, "Anesthetics and Other Medications."

Modification of the ECT Procedure

One of the most important aspects of the pre-ECT evaluation is to recommend appropriate modifications of the ECT procedure based on the medical history or physical findings. In patients with a skull defect (e.g., traumatic defect, craniotomy), electrode placement may need to be altered to accommodate the distorted anatomy. Also, identification of specific premedications for ECT may be noted in the pre-ECT evaluation.

Management of Medications

All medications that a patient takes should be reviewed as part of the pre-ECT evaluation for their possible roles in increasing the morbidity or decreasing the efficacy of ECT. Some commonly prescribed medications that are concerns are lithium, benzodiazepines, anticonvulsants, and theophylline. Evidence indicates that concomitant use of lithium and ECT may increase the risk of cognitive deficits, encephalopathy, and spontaneous seizures, although this has been disputed (Dolenc and Rasmussen 2005; Mukherjee 1993; Small and Milstein 1990).

Benzodiazepines or other anticonvulsants may raise the seizure threshold and decrease seizure efficacy. If the patient requires sedation, hydroxyzine or diphenhydramine is usually preferred over benzodiazepines. For a patient who is severely agitated, antipsychotic medications are preferred. Because the time required to safely taper a patient completely off benzodiazepines may be clinically prohibitive, some practitioners have administered the benzodiazepine antagonist flumazenil intravenously a few seconds following infusion of the anesthetic agent (Berigan et al. 1995). There is substantial concern regarding the effects of anticonvulsant agents on seizure threshold—that is, the ease with which seizures can be electrically induced—particularly given the increasingly frequent usage of these medications for patients with treatment-resistant major depression. However, there are some data suggesting that not all anticonvulsants have equivalent effects in this regard, with lamotrigine being less problematic than others (Sienaert and Peuskens 2007).

Most patients who are referred for ECT have unsuccessfully tried several psychiatric medications or combinations of medications. Although some practitioners discontinue any psychotropic medications prior to ECT, this is not always feasible because of the half-life of the medication or patients' special needs. In these cases, initiation of ECT should not be held back if the risk is low. Psychotropic medication use may be permitted during ECT for patients who are psychotic or severely agitated. These medications have been found to be particularly helpful to patients, and tolerability of ECT treatment was not influenced by the medications (Nothdurfter et al. 2006).

Some practitioners have suggested that concomitant psychopharmacotherapy may augment the therapeutic effect of ECT. However, limited data support this possibility, and only a few studies have shown an advantage of using a combination of ECT and tricyclic antidepressants (Baghai et al. 2006; Sackeim et al. 2009). Based on a modest-sized retrospective case series, Baghai et al. (2006) indicated that seizure duration was not affected by most antidepressants, although selective serotonin reuptake inhibitors (SSRIs) caused an overall lengthened seizure activity. Furthermore, the authors believed that a significant enhancement of therapeutic effectiveness could be seen in the patient group receiving tricyclics, SSRIs, or mirtazapine. In a more recent, large-scale prospective study, Sackeim et al. (2009) reported enhancement of ECT response with nortriptyline and, to a lesser degree, venlafaxine. They also found that while concomitant usage of nortriptyline was associated with diminished memory deficits with ECT, the opposite appeared to be the case with venlafaxine. Clearly, such provocative findings require corroboration.

The practitioner must also be very clear about which medications should be given the day of ECT and how they should be administered. The patient is usually allowed no food or drink after midnight prior to ECT. Any prescribed oral medications that exert a protective effect during ECT (e.g., antihypertensive, antiarrhythmic, analgesic, antireflux medications) can be given with sips of water at least 2 hours prior to ECT. If anticholinergic medication (e.g., glycopyrrolate or atropine) is prescribed to minimize secretions, it is usually administered intravenously at least 15 minutes prior to ECT. If it is being used to minimize parasympathetic cardiovascular effects, it is best given intravenously at the time of the treatment (see Chapter 6, "Anesthetics and Other Medications"). For patients with glaucoma, pretreatment with an ophthalmic beta-blocker preparation may prevent the rise in intraocular pressure by blunting the hypertensive response. In patients with asthma, chronic bronchitis, or chronic obstructive pulmonary disease, asthma inhalers that induce immediate bronchodilation should be considered prior to induction with general anesthesia.

Medications that prolong seizure duration must be considered with caution in the context of ECT. Although widespread use has diminished in the United States, theophylline increases the risk of prolonged seizures or even status epilepticus in ECT patients (Fink and Sackeim 1998).

Management of Special Medical Conditions

Cardiovascular Disease

The cardiovascular risk of ECT is a product of the stress of ECT itself (see Chapter 9, "Cardiovascular Response") and the severity and stability of coronary artery disease in the patient (Applegate 1997). Studies have indicated that patients with cardiac disease have a higher rate of cardiac complications during ECT than those without cardiac disease (Zielinski et al. 1993) and that the type of preexisting abnormality tends to predict the type of cardiac complication that occurs. Thus, post-ECT arrhythmias are correlated with the presence of pre-ECT arrhythmias (Huuhka et al. 2003). However, most cardiac complications are transitory and do not interrupt the completion of ECT.

Patients with hypertensive or coronary artery disease must be stabilized prior to initiating treatments (Weiner et al. 2000). Once stabilized, they should receive their medication prior to each treatment. Consideration should be given to the use of an acute sympatholytic during treatment in patients with coronary artery disease (see Chapter 6, "Anesthetics and Other Medications").

A retrospective study of patients with cardiac pacemakers who presented for ECT found that no extra precautions are needed other than routine electrocardiographic monitoring (MacPherson et al. 2006). Patients with cardiac pacemakers usually have a decreased likelihood of pathological arrhythmias due to the artificial pacing. A demand pacemaker may require conversion to a fixed mode at the time of treatment to prevent inappropriate activation. Similarly, some types of implanted defibrillators need to be noninvasively deactivated immediately before each treatment (Pinski and Trohman 1995). In both cases, advice of a cardiology consultant should be sought if uncertainty exists.

Diabetes

ECT is often performed on psychiatric patients who have diabetes. In patients with diabetes, glycemic control and insulin requirements usually show no changes over the course of treatment or after individual treatments (Rasmussen et al. 2006), although interindividual variation occurs. When changes are necessary, they are usually associated with changes in dietary or activity levels (Netzel et al. 2002). For the nondiabetic patient, studies have found that ECT has no clinically significant effect on blood sugar (Rasmussen and Ryan 2005).

Because patients are usually allowed no food or drink prior to each treatment, the antidiabetic medication regimen must be adjusted for the patient with diabetes (Finestone and Weiner 1984). In particular, insulin dosages may need to be reduced and/or split on ECT days. Preferably, patients requiring insulin should be treated as early in the day as possible. Many practitioners use an intravenous drip containing a glucose solution if the patient will have a prolonged wait before treatment or if the patient's diabetic control is brittle. Because hypoglycemia increases the metabolic risk of seizures, a fingerstick glucose level should be checked 30 minutes prior to each treatment.

Asthma

Because ECT requires the administration of general anesthesia, special care is needed for patients with asthma. Overall, however, ECT appears to be safe for patients with asthma. In a retrospective study of 34 patients with asthma who underwent ECT, Mueller et al. (2006) found that four (12%) experienced exacerbations of their asthma on a total of five occasions. Each exacerbation was successfully treated with standard therapy, and all patients completed their course of ECT. Because theophylline significantly increases the seizure duration and raises the risk of prolonged seizures (Rasmussen and Zorumski 1993), dosages should be minimized and blood levels checked prior to each ECT treatment, until stable values can be assured.

Epilepsy

Anticonvulsant agents are well recognized for making adequate seizure induction more difficult with ECT, although there is some evidence that this may not be the case with lamotrigine (Sienaert and Peuskens 2007). Still, limited data are available on the best clinical practice of ECT in patients with epilepsy. In general, dosages of anticonvulsants should be minimized, and the morning dose on the day of ECT should be delayed until after the treatment. Similar to the management of glucose levels, blood levels of anticonvulsants should be checked prior to ECT treatment until stable values can be assured. In a case series review of 43 patients with epilepsy treated with ECT, Lunde et al. (2006) found that the majority had adequate seizures during ECT without a reduction of the concomitant anticonvulsant dosage, although a few patients did require dosage reductions. The authors also observed that seven of the patients may have had spontaneous seizures during the treatment course, but the possibility of pseudoseizures or nonictal phenomena seemed quite likely in several of those cases.

Pregnancy

Pregnancy is not a contraindication to ECT, although an obstetrical consultation is recommended for every patient who is pregnant, and noninvasive fetal monitoring should be performed when indicated (Anderson and Reti 2009; Walker and Swartz 1994; Wisner and Perel 1998). The pharmacological agents used at the time of ECT have no known teratogenic or other adverse effects. However, during the last trimester, a greater risk of gastric reflux is possible due to the mass effect produced by the growing fetus.

Head Trauma

Patients with skull defects may require modified stimulus electrode placement to avoid a low-impedance path for the electrical current into the brain (see Chapter 4, "Basics").

Risk-Benefit Considerations

The decision to treat a patient with ECT is made after a careful risk-benefit analysis of ECT and alternative treatments. The diagnostic and strategic indications for ECT were discussed in Chapter 2, "Indications for Use." As stated there, even though ECT is typically used when patients have been refractory to or intolerant of psychotropic medications, it should not be viewed as a treatment of last resort. In some situations, ECT may be the initial treatment of choice (American Psychiatric Association 2001).

Writing the ECT Consultation

The ECT evaluation may be viewed as a second opinion if performed by a physician who is not the specific patient's primary inpatient or outpatient attending physician. Regardless of who performs the ECT evaluation, the report should adhere to salient features noted in this chapter. Chiefly, the decision to proceed with ECT can be supported by an ECT-responsive diagnosis and failure of other treatment modalities. If ECT is to be used as the primary treatment option, written justification of the rationale should be documented.

In addition to confirming the diagnosis and justifying ECT, the consulting physician should include in the report any specific ECT-related treatment plans. Electrode placement, modification of the patient's regular medication regimen, addition of pre-ECT medications or post-ECT medications, and issues related to anesthesia should be included. The report may also include an estimate of the approximate number of treatments. If ECT is not recommended, the ECT provider may suggest alternative treatment options that may not have been considered by the primary treatment team. Reference to the informed consent process should be made in the ECT evaluation, but the evaluation itself typically does not replace a more formal written informed consent.

Informed Consent

As for any invasive medical procedure (particularly one that involves general anesthesia), informed consent must be obtained for ECT (American Psychiatric Association 2001). Whereas psychiatrists routinely obtain verbal consent from patients prior to initiating pharmacological treatments, the standard for consent regarding invasive procedures in the United States requires written

Table 3–4.   Components of informed consent for ECT

- Information about benefits of treatment (including potential duration of effect)
- Information about risks (potential adverse effects) of treatment
- Information about alternatives to ECT
- Assessment of the patient's decision-making capacity

informed consent. Regulations concerning the informed consent process for ECT vary considerably from state to state. For example, in some jurisdictions, the consent form must include specific information identified by state regulations. The treating physician must be familiar with local jurisdictional requirements (Harris 2006).

For the consent to be deemed valid, it must meet four criteria (Table 3–4). The patient must be provided with information about risks and benefits, as well as alternative forms of treatment. The patient also must have the capacity to provide consent, and the consenter must make the decision him- or herself.

The informed consent for ECT should be obtained by a physician member of the ECT treatment team. A separate consent for the provision of general anesthesia should be obtained by the anesthesia team (i.e., the anesthesiologist or his or her designee).

Consent must always be obtained before the initial treatment in an index treatment course. Because continuation or maintenance ECT represents a separate treatment series, informed consent should be reobtained before its initiation and at least every 6 months thereafter, using a separate consent form, as the purpose of the maintenance treatment is generally prophylactic rather than therapeutic. ECT is unusual in that an index treatment course consists of a series of separate individual treatments that may span several weeks. Because the course is a series, consent for each treatment should not be necessary (except in rare cases where required by state law). However, both the patient and the physician should understand that informed consent is an ongoing process and that the consenter may withdraw consent for ECT at any time during the series.

Information about ECT should be presented not with the goal of merely obtaining a signature on a consent form, but rather to enable the consenter to make an informed decision. This process involves the physician presenting information to the consenter in a plain, comprehensible manner. Situations involving substantially increased risk or major treatment modifications should also be addressed, and such communications should be documented in the medical record.

Most states require that the formal consent materials provide a certain minimum amount of information. This information can be provided either in a single consent form or in two documents: a brief formal consent form (see examples in Appendix D) and a more lengthy patient information sheet (see example in Appendix C). The American Psychiatric Association has recommended that such materials cover nine general areas of patient information (American Psychiatric Association 2001):

1. A description of the ECT procedure (including the times the treatment is given, the location, and the typical number of treatments to be administered)
2. Why ECT is being recommended and by whom
3. Alternative treatment methods
4. A statement that any benefits may be transient
5. The likelihood and anticipated severity of major risks (mortality, cardiovascular complications, and cognitive changes) and common minor risks
6. A description of behavioral restrictions that may be necessary
7. An acknowledgment that consent for ECT is voluntary and can be withdrawn at any time
8. An offer to answer questions regarding the recommended treatment at any time and the name of the person to contact for such questions
9. A statement that consent for ECT also implies consent for delivery of any emergency medical or surgical interventions that become necessary (a very rare event) while the patient is unconscious

Some practitioners supplement the patient information materials described above with more detailed written documents and/or videotapes especially designed for educating patients. A listing of educational books and a videotape for patient education can be found in Appendix B.

Some data suggest that even elderly patients who are severely depressed often retain their ability to provide informed consent for ECT (Lapid et al. 2004). Patients should be considered to have the capacity to provide consent unless compelling evidence suggests otherwise. For such capacity to be present, a patient should be able to 1) comprehend the nature and seriousness of the illness for which treatment is being offered, 2) understand the information provided concerning the treatment modality, and 3) form and express a rational response based on this information. If the patient lacks capacity under these guidelines, informed consent must be provided via applicable state or federal statutes, often by a court-appointed guardian. In some jurisdictions, next of kin who have not been identified previously as proxy decision makers may not be able to provide informed consent for patients who lack such capacity. In complex circumstances, medicolegal support may be available from the hospital counsel's office or the psychiatrist's or hospital's medical malpractice risk management office.

Sample consent forms (for acute and maintenance/continuation ECT) are provided in Appendix D. These forms are meant to serve as a model that can be adapted to the specific needs of the region in which ECT is practiced.

References

American Psychiatric Association: The Practice of Electroconvulsive Therapy: Recommendations for Treatment, Training, and Privileging (A Task Force Report of the American Psychiatric Association), 2nd Edition. Washington, DC, American Psychiatric Publishing, 2001

Anderson EL, Reti IM: ECT in pregnancy: a review of the literature from 1941–2007. Psychosom Med 71:235–242, 2009

Applegate RJ: Diagnosis and management of ischemic heart disease in the patient scheduled to undergo electroconvulsive therapy. Convuls Ther 13:128–144, 1997

Baghai TC, Marcuse A, Brosch M, et al: The influence of concomitant antidepressant medication on safety, tolerability and clinical effectiveness of electroconvulsive therapy. World J Biol Psychiatry 7:82–90, 2006

Berigan TR, Harazin J, Williams HL: Use of flumazenil in conjunction with electroconvulsive therapy. Am J Psychiatry 152:957, 1995

Dolenc TJ, Rasmussen KG: The safety of electroconvulsive therapy and lithium in combination: a case series and review of the literature. J ECT 21:165–170, 2005

Edwards RM, Stoudemire A, Vela MA, et al: Intraocular pressure changes in nonglaucomatous patients undergoing electroconvulsive therapy. Convuls Ther 6:209–213, 1990

Finestone DH, Weiner RD: Effects of ECT on diabetes mellitus: an attempt to account for conflicting data. Acta Psychiatr Scand 70:321–326, 1984

Fink M, Sackeim HA: Theophylline and the risk of status epilepticus in ECT. J ECT 14:286–290, 1998

Harris V: Electroconvulsive therapy: administrative codes, legislation, and professional recommendations. J Am Acad Psychiatry Law 34:406–411, 2006

Huuhka MJ, Seinela L, Reinikainen P, et al: Cardiac arrythmias induced by ECT in elderly psychiatric patients: experience with 48-hour Holter monitoring. J ECT 19:22–25, 2003

Klapheke MM: Electroconvulsive therapy consultation: an update. Convuls Ther 13:227–241, 1997

Lapid MI, Rummans TA, Pankratz VS, et al: Decisional capacity of depressed elderly to consent to electroconvulsive therapy. J Geriatr Psychiatry Neurol 17:42–46, 2004

Lunde ME, Lee EK, Rasmussen KG: Electroconvulsive therapy in patients with epilepsy. Epilepsy Behav 9:355–359, 2006

MacPherson RD, Loo CK, Barrett N: Electroconvulsive therapy in patients with cardiac pacemakers. Anaesth Intensive Care 34:470–474, 2006

McCall WV, Minneman SA, Weiner RD, et al: Dental pathology in ECT patients prior to treatment. Convuls Ther 8:19–24, 1992

Minneman SA: A history of oral protection for the ECT patient: past, present, and future. Convuls Ther 11:94–103, 1995

Mueller PS, Schak KM, Barnes RD, et al: Safety of electroconvulsive therapy in patients with asthma. Neth J Med 64:417–421, 2006

Mukherjee S: Combined ECT and lithium therapy. Convuls Ther 9:274–284, 1993

Netzel PJ, Mueller PS, Rummans TA, et al: Safety, efficacy, and effects on glycemic control of electroconvulsive therapy in insulin-requiring type 2 diabetic patients. J ECT 18:16–21, 2002

Nothdurfter C, Eser D, Schule C, et al: The influence of concomitant neuroleptic medication on safety, tolerability and clinical effectiveness of electroconvulsive therapy. World J Biol Psychiatry 7:162–170, 2006

Pinski SL, Trohman RG: Implantable cardioverter-defibrillators: implications for the nonelectrophysiologist. Ann Intern Med 122:770–777, 1995

Porter RJ, Douglas K, Knight RG: Monitoring of cognitive effects during a course of electroconvulsive therapy: recommendations for clinical practice. J ECT 24:25–34, 2008

Rasmussen KG, Ryan DA: The effect of electroconvulsive therapy treatments on blood sugar in nondiabetic patients. J ECT 21:232–234, 2005

Rasmussen KG, Zorumski CF: Electroconvulsive therapy in patients taking theophylline. J Clin Psychiatry 54:427–431, 1993

Rasmussen KG, Karpyak VM, Hammill SC: Lack of effect of ECT on Holter monitor recordings before and after treatment. J ECT 20:45–47, 2004

Rasmussen KG, Ryan DA, Mueller PS: Blood glucose before and after ECT treatments in Type 2 diabetic patients. J ECT 22:124–126, 2006

Sackeim HA, Dillingham EM, Prudic J, et al: Effect of concomitant pharmacotherapy on electroconvulsive therapy outcomes. Arch Gen Psychiatry 66:729–737, 2009

Sienaert P, Peuskens J: Anticonvulsants during electroconvulsive therapy: review and recommendations. J ECT 23:120–123, 2007

Small JG, Milstein V: Lithium interactions: lithium and electroconvulsive therapy. J Clin Psychopharmacol 10:346–350, 1990

Takada JY, Solimene MC, da Luz PL, et al: Assessment of the cardiovascular effects of electroconvulsive therapy in individuals older than 50 years. Braz J Med Biol Res 38:1349–1357, 2005

Tess AV, Smetana GW: Medical evaluation of patients undergoing electroconvulsive therapy. N Engl J Med 360:1437–1444, 2009

Troup PJ, Small JG, Milstein V, et al: Effect of electroconvulsive therapy on cardiac rhythm, conduction and repolarization. Pacing Clin Electrophysiol 1:172–177, 1978

Walker R, Swartz CM: Electroconvulsive therapy during high-risk pregnancy. Gen Hosp Psychiatry 16:348–353, 1994

Weiner RD, Coffey CE, Krystal AD: Electroconvulsive therapy in the medical and neurologic patient, in Psychiatric Care of the Medical Patient, 2nd Edition. Edited by Stoudemire A, Fogel BS, Greenberg D. New York, Oxford University Press, 2000, pp 419–428

Wisner KL, Perel JM: Psychopharmacologic agents and electroconvulsive therapy during pregnancy and the puerperium, in Psychiatric Consultation in Childbirth Settings: Parent- and Child-Oriented Approaches. Edited by Cohen RL. New York, Plenum, 1998, pp 165–206

Zielinski RJ, Roose SP, Devanand DP, et al: Cardiovascular complications of ECT in depressed patients with cardiac disease. Am J Psychiatry 150:904–909, 1993

PART 2

Electrical Stimulus and Procedure

4

Basics

Richard D. Weiner, M.D., Ph.D.

The goal of the physician during ECT is to deliver an electrical stimulus large enough to induce an adequate seizure while minimizing the risk of significant side effects. This seizure initiation occurs via a massive synchronous recruitment of certain intracerebral neuronal centers, as occurs in spontaneous major motor seizures. The electrical stimulus can be delivered in a number of ways utilizing different modes of delivery, stimulus types, and stimulus intensities. The physician has to determine what electrical dose to administer to each individual patient to assure a safe and effective treatment. A simple understanding of a few basic concepts concerning the electrical stimulus is important to this decision.

Electrical Waveforms Used With ECT

The electrical stimulus can be delivered via a variety of waveforms. A waveform is the "shape" of the stimulus as a function of time. Historically, the two most commonly used waveforms in ECT are the sine wave and brief pulse waveforms (Sackeim et al. 1994), which are depicted in Figure 4–1.

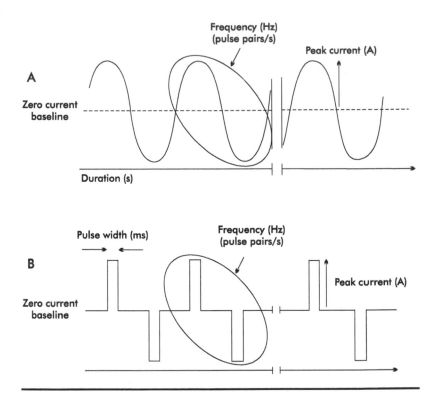

Figure 4–1.   Sine wave (A) and brief pulse (B) waveforms.

Sine Wave ECT

When Cerletti and Bini began experimenting with the induction of seizures by electricity (see Chapter 1, "History of Electroconvulsive Therapy," and Shorter and Healy 2007), they used, as a matter of convenience, the waveform that is supplied by wall outlets: the sine wave. Sine wave currents are characterized by a continuous stream of electricity that flows in alternating directions. The number of alterations in direction, or cycles of negative and positive current flow, is referred to as the frequency of the stimulus and is measured in hertz (Hz), defined as the number of cycles per second. In the United States, standard wall current consists of a 60-Hz sine wave, which means that 60 positive and 60 negative departures from the baseline occur each second that the overall stimulus is being delivered.

Brief Pulse ECT

Beginning in the late 1970s, the brief pulse waveform replaced the sine wave stimulus in ECT in most countries. Like the sine wave stimulus, the brief pulse waveform is bidirectional (i.e., has alternating positive and negative phases). However, as opposed to the continuously undulating sine wave, the brief pulse consists of a series of instantaneously rising and falling rectangular pulses of current, with adjacent pulses separated by brief periods of no electrical activity (see Figure 4–1).

Brief pulses are characterized by four stimulus parameters: pulse width, frequency, duration, and peak current (see Figure 4–1). The duration of each pulse is referred to as the *pulse width,* which is measured in milliseconds (ms; thousandths of a second). *Pulse frequency,* by convention, is defined in terms of pulse pairs per second, although it is common practice to use the same unit of measure, hertz, as used for the sine wave. The actual number of pulses per second is twice the frequency. In the example shown in Figure 4–1B, a brief pulse frequency of 60 Hz would be associated with 60 positive and 60 negative departures from the baseline each second during the passage of the stimulus. *Duration* is defined as the length of the entire series of pulses delivered, and is measured in seconds. It is functionally the same as the time elapsed between the first and last pulse in the series. The final stimulus parameter is *peak current,* which is the maximum intensity of each pulse, measured from the zero baseline, in amperes.

Ultra-Brief Pulse ECT

Beginning in the late 1990s, renewed interest has been shown in the so-called ultra-brief stimulus waveform (Loo et al. 2007; Pisvejc et al. 1998; Sackeim et al. 2008). Operationally, a "brief" pulse has a pulse width of 0.5–2.0 ms, whereas the width of an "ultra-brief" pulse is less than 0.5 ms. (The clinical implications of pulse width are discussed in Chapter 5, "Clinical Applications.")

The Electrical Stimulus

Seizure Threshold

Seizure threshold is the total amount of electricity necessary to induce a seizure and, as discussed in Chapter 5, "Clinical Applications," is a parameter that is integral to stimulus dosing in clinical practice. The physiological efficiency of the brief pulse stimulus in activating brain neurons is more optimal than the sine wave because of its rapid rise and fall. In that regard, its relatively short "on" time is analogous to that of endogenous neuroelectrical signals within the brain—that is, action potentials. For this reason, evoking a generalized seizure using a brief pulse device typically requires much less overall stimulus intensity than does a sine wave stimulus. Theoretically, a similar situation should exist in regard to ultra-brief pulses versus brief pulses, with the ultra-brief pulses being even more efficient in terms of neuronal excitation, and thereby associated with a lower seizure threshold than brief pulses.

Current, Voltage, and Impedance

All electrical signals can be characterized by three primary variables: current, voltage, and impedance. In a physical sense, *current* is the number of electrons per second flowing through a circuit. In this case, the circuit is made up of the ECT machine, the stimulus cables, the stimulus electrodes, and the patient's head. *Voltage* is the force that drives the flow of electrons during the stimulus. It is the push of the system. *Impedance* is a measure of the obstacle to the current flow. It is the level of resistance to be overcome. In ECT, the terms *impedance* and *resistance* can be used interchangeably, because other factors potentially involved in impedance—that is, capacitance and inductance—are not major contributors in ECT. The greater the resistance (or impedance), the greater the push (or voltage) required for the fixed flow of electrons. In practical terms, a higher resistance is most often encountered in ECT with poor stimulus electrode contact, which requires a higher voltage to deliver a given current level. Conversely, the lower the impedance, the less push or voltage required to move a fixed current. The relationship among current, voltage, and resistance is called Ohm's law and is expressed in the equation

$$current = voltage / resistance$$

where current is measured in amperes (A) or milliamperes (mA), voltage is measured in volts (V), and resistance (impedance) is measured in ohms (Ω).

Mode of Stimulus Delivery

In addition to the type of waveform used, ECT devices differ in whether they administer the stimulus via a *constant current* or *constant voltage*. If we apply Ohm's law to the administration of the electrical stimulus, we find that ECT devices must allow the user to set either current (constant-current device) or voltage (constant-voltage device). In either case, the other measure of intensity varies with resistance, according to Ohm's law. Because current is now recognized as being of greater physiological importance than voltage in ECT, constant-current devices are preferable because they allow the user a greater control over stimulus intensity.

In other words, with a constant-current device, such as the ECT machines presently marketed in the United States, the practitioner predetermines the amount of current the patient will receive (e.g., 800 mA). Using the above equation for Ohm's law, the actual amount of current delivered (in milliamperes) would theoretically remain fixed, with any variation in impedance (ohms) being reflected by a proportional change in voltage while the current remains fixed. As an example, a doubling in impedance from 150 Ω to 300 Ω would not affect the amount of current (800 mA) delivered. However, again using Ohm's law, the voltage would also double from 120 V to 240 V. In practice, the ability of constant-current ECT devices to maintain current at a constant level breaks down when the impedance is grossly elevated (e.g., due to extremely poor stimulus electrode contact). In such cases, the devices limit voltage output as a safety feature (discussed in the following section).

Practical Considerations Regarding Impedance

As is evident in the previous discussion, the electrical impedance during the passage of the stimulus current is a very important measure. It can differ substantially across patients, and it can vary from treatment to treatment in the same patient (Coffey et al. 1995; Sackeim et al. 1991, 1994).

The primary source of impedance, as monitored during an ECT treatment, is the scalp tissue that underlies the stimulus electrodes. Because the skull is associated with extremely high intrinsic impedance, most of the electrical stimulus current is shunted across the scalp tissues between the electrodes without ever passing through the brain. As a result, only a fraction of the stimulus current actually enters the brain unless a low-impedance pathway to the brain exists (e.g., a skull defect). For this reason, stimulus electrodes should never be placed over or adjacent to a defect.

Because of the current's shunting across the scalp, the amount of current entering the skull is much less than that present at the stimulus electrodes. In addition, this lower amount of current is spread over a large surface area, so that the current density—that is, the amount of current per square centimeter—is further diminished. The electrical stimulus is attenuated even further during its passage through the skull, because of the large voltage drop that takes place across that structure's high impedance. All of these effects result in the fact that at the level of the brain substance itself, both current intensity and voltage are markedly lower than at the stimulus electrodes, such that a much weaker electrical current passes through neurons. This fact should not be surprising because sometimes even a high-intensity stimulus delivered by the ECT device is insufficient to induce the level of neuronal activation necessary to generate seizure activity.

A too-low scalp impedance (e.g., 100 Ω) is associated with an increased scalp shunting of current, a lower proportion of current entering the brain, and therefore diminished effectiveness in producing a seizure. This situation can occur when the ECT electrodes are placed too close together or when a conducting medium, such as sweat, saline, or electrode gel, forms a low-impedance pathway (short circuit) between the electrodes. More commonly, the impedance is too high. This situation can occur when the stimulus electrodes are in poor contact with the skin, causing the current to flow through a much smaller area. Because of the associated voltage limiting by the device, this situation also makes it less likely that an effective stimulus will be delivered and raises the theoretical risk of a skin burn (although this would be extremely unlikely with present devices). Table 4–1 summarizes the causes of variations in impedance.

To estimate whether impedance during the passage of the stimulus current will be too high or too low, brief pulse devices in the United States incorporate a self-test procedure. This feature involves the passage of a very low current through the entire electrical circuit pertinent to ECT (i.e., cable, leads, electrodes, and patient), allowing an estimation of impedance prior to stimulation. This low current is well below the patient's perceptual threshold, even if fully awake and alert. The impedance to this small current is typically much greater than that encountered during the actual stimulus. This difference is due to the fact that the impedance of the scalp tissue underlying the stimulus electrode is voltage sensitive and drops virtually instantaneously during the passage of the stimulus current. For this reason, the impedance during the stimulus current is termed the *dynamic* impedance (relating to the change that occurs during the passage of the stimulus current), and the impedance during the self-test procedure is termed the *static* impedance (reflecting the

Table 4–1. Cause of variations in impedance

Causes of high impedance	Causes of low impedance
Poor contact of electrodes with scalp	Stimulus electrodes are too close together
Poor preparation of scalp	Low impedance pathway (sweat, conducting gel)
Faulty connection of electrodes	

baseline impedance state). Typical dynamic impedance is around 220 Ω (range 120–350 Ω), whereas typical static impedance is approximately 350–2,000 Ω for most devices (range 300–3,000 Ω). Impedances are higher for women than for men and greater for unilateral stimulus electrode placement than for bilateral placement (Coffey et al. 1995). Because impedance is also inversely proportional to stimulus electrode size (surface area in contact with the scalp), impedances are lower in the United States, where ECT devices have stimulus electrodes 2 inches in diameter, than in some other countries where stimulus electrodes are smaller.

As noted earlier, a frequent cause of markedly elevated stimulus intensity is inadequate coupling of the stimulus electrodes to the scalp (caused, e.g., by insufficient preparation of the scalp; insufficient use of electrode gel, particularly when hair is in the way; or too little pressure in the application of the stimulus electrodes to the scalp). Another cause of very high static impedance is the failure to connect the stimulus cable to the stimulus electrodes or the loss of such a connection. If the static impedance is too high (e.g., >3,000 Ω with the Somatics Thymatron® System IV and DGx [http://www.thymatron.com] or MECTA spECTrum [http://www.mectacorp.com] ECT devices, or "failure" with the MECTA SR and JR devices), the electrode cables and the electrode application should be checked. The static impedance should then be retested to ensure safe treatment. The MECTA spECTrum provides a continuous and automatic determination of static impedance, whereas the Thymatron® devices and the MECTA SR and JR devices require manual triggering of the static impedance measurement. Therefore, the self-test procedure with the latter devices should be assessed near in time to actual stimulus delivery (although additional testing prior to that time is often performed to ensure that the static impedance is within range at baseline).

Total Amount of Electricity Delivered With ECT: Charge and Energy

For various reasons, being able to describe the total amount of stimulus intensity delivered, in the form of a single composite intensity measure, is desirable. Such a measure, for example, will allow overall stimulus dose to be represented by a single number. Two such composite measures are charge and energy, both of which are automatically calculated by the present generation of U.S. ECT devices. The first of these measures, *charge*, represents the product of the amount of current in a single pulse and the number of pulses delivered in the series, and is measured in millicoulombs (mC). The amount of current in a single pulse is the product of peak current (in amperes) and pulse width (in milliseconds), whereas the number of pulses is the product of twice the frequency (in hertz) and duration (in seconds).

As an example, if one has a stimulus characterized by 0.5-ms pulses of 0.8-A intensity and a frequency of 70 Hz, delivered for a duration of 3 seconds, the charge is $0.5 \times 0.8 \times 2 \times 70 \times 3 = 168$ mC.

Energy, in the context of ECT stimulus dose, is defined as the product of voltage and current over the entire stimulus duration. With a constant-current ECT device, using Ohm's law to replace voltage with the product of current and dynamic impedance, it becomes clear that energy is proportional to dynamic impedance. Because dynamic impedance is not known until after passage of the stimulus, energy, as opposed to charge, is not predictable prior to the stimulus. For this and other reasons, charge is the preferred means of expressing total stimulus dosage.

Device characteristics, stimulus parameter ranges, and maximum output charge and energy (assuming a dynamic impedance of 220 Ω) are given in Table 4–2 for the present generation of ECT devices made in the United States as of December 2008. Figure 4–2 provides photographs of examples of these devices. Each of these devices provides the user with a printout of the pertinent electrical output information regarding the ECT stimulus, including both static and dynamic impedance.

Table 4–2. Specifications of ECT devices used in the United States (as of January 2009)

	MECTA				Somatics		
Specification	SR-1 and JR-1[a]	SR-2 and JR-2[a]	spECTrum 5000Q/4000Q[b]	spECTrum 5000M/4000M[b]	Thymatron® DGx[a]	Thymatron® DGx with FlexDial[a,c]	Thymatron® System IV[b]
Peak current (mA)	500–800	800	500–800	800	900	900	900
Frequency (pulse pairs per second)	40–90	70	20–120	20–120	30–70	30–70	10–140
Pulse width (ms)	0.5–2.0	0.5–4.0	0.3–2.0	0.3–2.0	1.0	0.5–1.5	0.25–1.5
Duration (seconds)	0.5–2.0	0.5–4.0	0.5–8.0	0.2–8.0	0.5–4.0	0.1–8.0	0.1–8.0
Charge[d] (mC)	20–576	20–576	5–576	6–576	27–504	25–504	25–504
Energy[d,e] (J)	2.2–101	13–101	1–101	1–101	5–99	5–99	5–99
EEG monitoring	SR-1 yes JR-1 no	SR-2 yes JR-2 no	5000Q yes 4000Q no	5000M yes 4000M no	Yes	Yes	Yes
Computer monitoring and storage capability	No	No	Yes	Yes	Yes	Yes	Yes

Note. EEG=electroencephalogram; J=joules; mA=milliamperes; mC=millicoulombs; ms=milliseconds.
[a]Manufacturer's second-generation device.
[b]Manufacturer's third-generation device.
[c]Optional.
[d]At time of writing, maximum device output charge in the United States for both U.S. ECT device manufacturers are limited by the Food and Drug Administration to what is shown in this table. For some other countries, these companies' devices are available with extended stimulus parameter ranges, allowing for approximately double the maximum output charge.
[e]Energy values assume a dynamic impedance of 220 Ω.

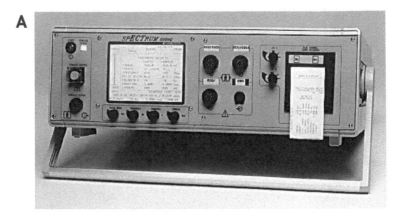

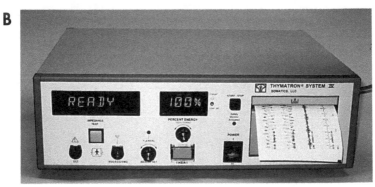

Figure 4–2. Photographs of ECT devices used in the United States: (A) The MECTA spECTrum 5000Q. (B) The Thymatron® System IV, courtesy of Somatics, LLC.

References

Coffey CE, Lucke J, Weiner RD, et al: Seizure threshold in electroconvulsive therapy, I: initial seizure threshold. Biol Psychiatry 37:713–720, 1995

Loo C, Sheehan P, Pigot M, et al: A report on mood and cognitive outcomes with right unilateral ultrabrief pulsewidth (0.3 ms) ECT and retrospective comparison with standard pulsewidth right unilateral ECT. J Affect Disord 103:277–281, 2007

Pisvejc J, Hyrman V, Sikora J, et al: A comparison of brief and ultrabrief pulse stimuli in unilateral ECT. J ECT 14:68–75, 1998

Sackeim HA, Devanand DP, Prudic J: Stimulus intensity, seizure threshold, and seizure duration: impact on the efficacy and safety of electroconvulsive therapy. Psychiatr Clin North Am 14:803–843, 1991

Sackeim HA, Long J, Luber B, et al: Physical properties and quantification of the ECT stimulus, I: basic principles. Convuls Ther 10:93–123, 1994

Sackeim HA, Prudic J, Nobler MS, et al: Effects of pulse width and electrode placement on the efficacy and cognitive effects of electroconvulsive therapy. Brain Stimulation 1:71–83, 2008

Shorter E, Healy D: Shock Therapy: A History of Electroconvulsive Treatment in Mental Illness. Piscataway, NJ, Rutgers University Press, 2007

5

Clinical Applications

Richard D. Weiner, M.D., Ph.D.

In Chapter 4, "Basics," I discussed the nature of the electrical stimulus in ECT and how the stimulus is characterized in terms of specific parameters. In this chapter, I discuss how the stimulus dose is chosen for clinical use. Topics include seizure adequacy, stimulus intensity, stimulus dosing strategies, and electrode placement.

Stimulus Dosing

As noted in Chapter 4, the purpose of the electrical stimulus in ECT is to generate an intracerebral current flow sufficient to induce an adequate generalized seizure within the brain. The seizure threshold is the minimum amount of stimulus electrical charge that will evoke such a response in a given patient at a given point in time. How a series of seizures produces the therapeutic effect of ECT is still unclear, but four important points are generally believed to be true:

1. An induced generalized seizure appears to be necessary for the production of a therapeutic response.

2. Seizures produced by barely suprathreshold stimuli are diminished in efficacy regardless of seizure duration, particularly with unilateral ECT (Sackeim et al. 1987). This effect is probably even more prominent with ultra-brief-pulse stimuli.
3. Seizures produced using markedly suprathreshold levels of stimulus intensity appear to be associated with increased cognitive side effects.
4. The stimulus intensity necessary to produce a therapeutically adequate seizure increases across subsequent treatments within an index ECT course.

These points are used to guide stimulus dosage based on the understanding of two parameters, seizure adequacy and stimulus intensity, discussed below.

Seizure Adequacy

For many years, an ECT treatment was considered therapeutically adequate if the seizure was generalized and of a certain duration (Abrams 2002; American Psychiatric Association 2001; Ottosson 1960). Typical recommended minimal durations have been 20–25 seconds for the motor response and 25 seconds for the ictal electroencephalographic (EEG) response. Because seizures tend to be shorter in elderly patients and also to diminish over the treatment course (Sackeim et al. 1991), some practitioners have used a lower criterion (e.g., <20-second seizure duration late in the treatment course if the patient is older than age 60 years). Seizure duration also may be affected by a number of other parameters, including the dose of anesthetic agent and the amount to which the stimulus exceeds the seizure threshold.

The precise minimum duration of the seizure required for optimal therapeutic effect has never been established, and data supporting specific criteria are not compelling, either in terms of the duration of an individual seizure or cumulative seizure duration over the entire treatment course. For this reason, the determination of treatment adequacy has been based on clinical outcome rather than on the number of seconds of seizure activity. As will be shown later in this chapter, there is also evidence that more intense stimuli sometimes lead to shorter, rather than longer, seizures, because of the nonlinear relationship between stimulus intensity and seizure duration (Frey et al. 2001). More recently, some evidence has indicated that other features of the seizure besides duration—for example, ictal EEG amplitude, pattern, and extent of postictal suppression—may offer promise as measures of seizure adequacy and thereby serve as guides to stimulus dosing (Azuma et al. 2007; Krystal et al. 1998, 2000; Mayur 2006; Perera et al. 2004) (see Chapter 8, "Ictal Electroencephalographic Response").

Stimulus Intensity

Evidence suggests that the greater the ECT stimulus intensity is with respect to seizure threshold (i.e., the more suprathreshold the stimulus), the more effective the treatments and the speedier the recovery (Sackeim et al. 1993). However, a higher stimulus intensity is directly related to an increase in cognitive side effects. Thus, the logical approach would be to deliver a stimulus that is moderately suprathreshold. Unfortunately, this solution is complex, for several reasons.

Seizure threshold varies greatly from person to person (up to 40-fold) and also from treatment to treatment, increasing variably over the treatment course (Sackeim et al. 1991). A number of factors influence an individual's seizure threshold (see Table 5–1), including age, gender, anesthetic agents, psychotropic medications, stimulus electrode placement, and the number and recency of previous ECT treatments.

Researchers do not yet know how much the stimulus needs to be above seizure threshold to be considered moderate, although for brief pulse bilateral ECT, the estimate is 50%–100% above the individual's seizure threshold (equivalent to 1.5–2 times seizure threshold), whereas for brief pulse unilateral ECT, estimates run 150%–500% above seizure threshold (i.e., 2.5–6 times seizure threshold). There is reason to believe that stimulus intensity needs to be greater than with brief pulse ECT for both unilateral and bilateral electrode placement, although sufficient information to specify a precise range does not presently exist. The stimulus dosing strategies described in the following section represent attempts to deal with this unresolved issue.

Stimulus Dosing Strategies

Two types of methods are generally used to determine electrical stimulus intensity: the dose-titration method and the preselected-dose method (American Psychiatric Association 2001). A third type of dosing strategy, EEG-based

Table 5–1. Factors influencing seizure threshold

Factor	Raises seizure threshold	Lowers seizure threshold
Age	Old	Young
Gender	Male	Female
Medication	Benzodiazepines	Pentylenetetrazol
	Anticonvulsants	Vasopressin
	Barbiturates	Benzodiazepine or alcohol withdrawal[a]
		Amphetamines
		Tricyclic antidepressants[a]
		Phenothiazines[a]
		Lithium[a]
		Reserpine
Brain disease	Diffuse, nonirritative[a]	Irritative[a]
Electrode placement	Bilateral, bifrontal[a] (requires more stimulus charge)	Unilateral (requires less stimulus charge)
Electrode contact	Poor contact[a]	Good contact[a]
Seizure activity	Seizure within last few days (standard ECT schedule)	

[a]Evidence is suggestive or theoretical but not conclusive.

dosing, has been proposed (Krystal and Weiner 1994; Krystal et al. 2000) but is still limited in its application.

Dose Titration

The dose-titration method allows the seizure threshold to be estimated at the first treatment. Stimulus dosing is then carried out with respect to that estimate at successive treatments. This technique involves starting with a stimulus dose at the first treatment that has a moderate (e.g., 50%) chance of inducing a seizure. Although beginning at a very low dose would theoretically allow a more precise estimate of seizure threshold for patients with low seizure thresholds, it would also result in excessive numbers of restimulations in patients with higher seizure thresholds. Taking into account some of the known relationships between seizure threshold and the factors of gender, electrode placement, and age, a dosing schedule can be developed that minimizes the number of restimulations required at the first treatment but at the same time allows a reasonably accurate estimate of initial seizure threshold. Sample schedules for ECT devices currently used in the United States, based on clinical experience at Duke University Medical Center with brief pulse stimuli (Coffey et al. 1995), are provided in Tables 5–2 through 5–4; general instructions for the use of the schedules in these three tables are listed in Table 5–5. It should be noted that these dosing protocols may differ from those included in device user manuals, which themselves tend to be empirically rather than scientifically based.

Separate dose titration schedules and instructions for ultra-brief-pulse stimuli are provided in Tables 5–6 through 5–8. Since very few data regarding stimulus dosing for ultra-brief-pulse exist at the time of this writing, the reader should be aware that the schedules reflected in these three tables are based on both extrapolation from clinical experience with brief-pulse stimulus dosing and theoretical modeling. Again, these schedules may differ from those contained in device user manuals.

Table 5–2.   Dose titration techniques for MECTA SR and JR models (brief-pulse stimuli)

Dose level	MECTA SR-1/JR-1					MECTA SR-2/JR-2	
	PW (msec)	F (/sec)	D (sec)	I (amp)	Charge (mcoul)	Energy level[a]	Charge (mcoul)
1[b]	1.0	40	0.50	0.8	32	1.0[c]	58
2[d]	1.0	40	0.75	0.8	48	1.0	58
3[e]	1.0	40	1.25	0.8	80	1.5	86
4	1.0	40	2.00	0.8	128	2.5	144
5	1.0	60	2.00	0.8	192	3.5	202
6	1.0	90	2.00	0.8	288	5.0	288
7	1.4	90	2.00	0.8	403	7.0	403
8	2.0	90	2.00	0.8	576	10.0	576

Note.   Pulse width, frequency, duration, and current are all adustable.
amp = amperes; mcoul = millicoulombs; msec = milliseconds; sec = seconds; /sec = Hertz.
[a]Actually proportional to maximum output charge, where a setting of 1 = 10% maximum output charge, and a setting of 10 = 100% of maximum output charge.
[b]Start at dose level 1 for unilateral ECT in female patients.
[c]Settings below this level may be associated with too brief a stimulus duration to induce seizures.
[d]Start at dose level 2 for bilateral ECT in female patients or unilateral ECT in male patients.
[e]Start at dose level 3 for bilateral ECT in male patients.

Table 5–3. Dose titration techniques for MECTA SpECTrum models (brief-pulse stimuli)

Dose level	MECTA SpECTrum 4000Q/5000Q					MECTA SpECTrum 4000M/5000M	
	PW (msec)	F (/sec)	D (sec)	I (amp)	Charge (mcoul)	Stimulus level[a] (%)	Charge (mcoul)
1[b]	1.0	40	0.50	0.8	32	5	29
2[c]	1.0	40	0.75	0.8	48	10	58
3[d]	1.0	40	1.25	0.8	80	15	86
4	1.0	40	2.00	0.8	128	25	144
5	1.0	60	2.00	0.8	192	35	202
6	1.0	60	3.00	0.8	288	50	288
7	1.0	60	4.50	0.8	432	70	403
8	1.0	60	6.00	0.8	576	100	576

Note. amp=amperes; mcoul=millicoulombs; msec=milliseconds; sec=seconds; /sec=Hertz.
[a]Percent of maximum output charge.
[b]Start at dose level 1 for unilateral ECT in female patients.
[c]Start at dose level 2 for bilateral ECT in female patients or unilateral ECT in male patients.
[d]Start at dose level 3 for bilateral ECT in male patients.

With these schedules, the dose at the first treatment is set according to the patient's gender and the stimulus electrode placement used (i.e., unilateral or bilateral), because some evidence indicates that these two factors account for more of the variance in seizure threshold than does age (Sackeim et al. 1991). If an adequate seizure is not obtained in response to the initial stimulus, the patient is restimulated after a short delay (generally less than 15 seconds) at a one-step increase of roughly 50% in overall intensity (charge). (Although smaller increments between steps lead to more precise estimates of seizure threshold, they also result in a higher number of restimulations. The 50% figure represents what I believe to be a reasonable compromise.) If an adequate seizure is still not elicited, the patient should be restimulated at a further one-step increment after an identical short delay. This process may be repeated for up to a total of four stimulations at the first treatment, except that a two-step increase should be used for the fourth stimulus to maximize the likelihood of achieving an adequate seizure. On average, only one restimulation is necessary at the first treatment (Coffey et al. 1995).

Table 5–4. Dose titration techniques for Somatics Thymatron DGx and System IV models (brief-pulse stimuli)

| Dose level | Thymatron DGx | | Thymatron System IV | |
	Energy level[a] (%)	Charge (mcoul)	Energy level[a] (%)	Charge (mcoul)
1[b]	5	25	5	25
2[c]	10[d]	50	10[d]	50
3[e]	15	76	15	76
4	25	75	25	75
5	35	115	35	115
6	50	173	50	173
7	70	259	70	259
8	100	403	100	403

Note. mcoul = millicoulombs.
[a]Percent of maximum output charge.
[b]Start at dose level 1 for unilateral ECT in female patients.
[c]Start at dose level 2 for bilateral ECT in female patients or unilateral ECT in male patients.
[d]Steps constrained to units of 5%.
[e]Start at dose level 3 for bilateral ECT in male patients.

The stimulus intensity that was successful in producing a seizure at the first treatment constitutes the estimate of the patient's seizure threshold at the beginning of the ECT course. The stimulus for successive treatments is then increased by at least one step (approximately 1.5 times the initial threshold) for bilateral ECT and three steps (approximately 3.4 times the initial threshold) for unilateral ECT, to be sufficiently above seizure threshold to ensure adequate and rapid treatment efficacy. As long as seizures appear adequate (see Chapter 8), the stimulus is kept at this level. Some practitioners choose to increase to as much as 6 times seizure threshold (McCall et al. 2000; Sackeim et al. 2000), but evidence to support such high levels (which may have cognitive ramifications) is not conclusive.

Unfortunately, because seizure threshold increases to a variable degree and at a variable rate over the ECT course, seizures are eventually missed or are inadequate in a high proportion of patients. When such an event occurs, an additional one-step (1.5 times) increment in stimulus intensity is indicated; some practitioners recommend a larger increase (e.g., two steps, or 2.25 times)

Table 5–5. Instructions for use of brief-pulse dose titration schedules shown in Tables 5–2 through 5–4

Threshold determination	1.	Start at level indicated by gender and electrode placement.
	2.	Increase level **one step** if restimulation is necessary.
	3.	If no adequate seizure has occurred after three stimulations at the first session (uncommon), jump **two levels** for the fourth stimulus.
	4.	If no adequate seizure has taken place after four stimulations at the first session (rare), abort the treatment session and go **one level** higher for initial stimulus at the second treatment session to continue titration.
Successive treatments	1.	After establishing lowest threshold level needed to produce an adequate seizure, **increase three steps** for the next treatment with *unilateral* ECT and **one step** with *bilateral* ECT.
	2.	Whenever any further increase in stimulus intensity is indicated because of a missed, abortive, or inadequate seizure (see Chapters 8 and 11), use **one- or two-step** increments for *unilateral* ECT and **one-step** increments for *bilateral* ECT.

with unilateral ECT. Because the rise in seizure threshold is not predictable, a minority of practitioners retitrate the stimulus dose for the patient at a later point in the ECT course (e.g., at the sixth treatment), whereas some others routinely increase the stimulus intensity intermittently (e.g., at every third treatment).

In this regard, the use of seizure duration as the primary measure of ensuring that the stimulus remains sufficiently suprathreshold (see Chapter 8 and Chapter 11, "Managing the ECT Seizure") is problematic, given that the complex relationship between relative stimulus intensity—that is, the extent to which a stimulus exceeds seizure threshold—and seizure duration is nonlinear. As shown in Figure 5–1, when the stimulus is barely suprathreshold, increasing stimulus intensity will be associated with a longer seizure duration. However, when the stimulus greatly exceeds seizure threshold, seizure duration can be expected to fall rather than increase. In addition, as the number of index ECT treatments increases, seizure threshold rises and seizure dura-

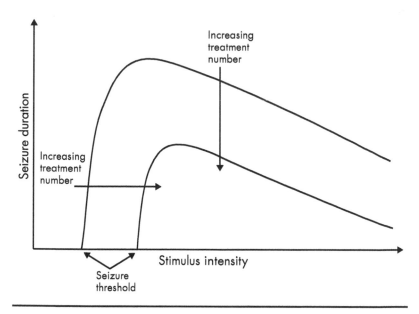

Figure 5–1. Effects of increasing treatment number on the relationship between stimulus intensity and seizure duration.

tion falls, resulting in a shift to the right and downward of the curve depicting the relationship between stimulus intensity and seizure duration. What this means is that some seizures that appear very brief may actually be associated with a higher relative stimulus intensity than longer seizures, particularly toward the end of an index ECT course. In practical terms, if increasing stimulus intensity is seen to lead to a decrease in seizure duration, that effect is evidence that the stimulus was well above seizure threshold.

There has been some concern that with unilateral brief-pulse (and both unilateral and bilateral ultra-brief-pulse) ECT, the barely suprathreshold seizure induced at the first treatment using the dose titration technique may be suboptimal from an efficacy standpoint (although this point remains to be proven). One option, though technically complex, is to induce a second, moderately suprathreshold seizure during the initial session of anesthesia. Because of the postictal refractory period, this technique requires waiting 2 minutes following completion of the initial EEG seizure before inducing the second seizure.

Table 5–6.   Dose titration techniques for MECTA SpECTrum models (ultra-brief-pulse stimuli)

| Dose level | MECTA SpECTrum 4000Q/5000Q | | | | | MECTA SpECTrum 4000M/5000M | |
	PW (msec)	F (/sec)	D (sec)	I (amp)	Charge (mcoul)	Stimulus level[a] (%)	Charge (mcoul)
1[b]	0.3	20	2.0	0.8	20	3	17
2[c]	0.3	30	2.0	0.8	29	5	29
3[d]	0.3	40	2.5	0.8	48	8	46
4	0.3	50	3.0	0.8	72	13	75
5	0.3	50	4.5	0.8	108	20	115
6	0.3	60	6.0	0.8	173	30	173
7	0.3	90	6.0	0.8	259	45	259
8	0.3	100	8.0	0.8	384	70	403
9	0.37	120	8.0	0.8	568	100	576

Note.   amp=amperes; mcoul=millicoulombs; msec=milliseconds; sec=seconds; /sec=Hertz.
[a]Percent of maximum output charge.
[b]Start at dose level 1 for unilateral ECT in female patients.
[c]Start at dose level 2 for bilateral ECT in female patients or unilateral ECT in male patients.
[d]Start at dose level 3 for bilateral ECT in male patients.

During this time period, it is essential to carefully monitor the patient for evidence that the effects of the anesthetic or muscle relaxant are wearing off, and to add an additional partial dose of either should that occur. For obvious reasons, one would not want to administer a higher anesthetic dosage initially, but one can administer an initial muscle relaxant dose that is 1.5 times what one would utilize otherwise. As noted above, this technique is technically challenging and should only be used by those with substantial experience with traditional dose titration.

Preselected Dose

The preselected dose is the second type of strategy for stimulus delivery. In its most crude form, often referred to as the *fixed-dose paradigm,* all patients receive the same stimulus dose, regardless of patient characteristics (McCall et al. 1995), usually at a relatively high level (e.g., 50%–100% of the device's maximum output intensity). This technique does not make any attempt to

Table 5–7. Dose titration technique for Somatics Thymatron System IV model (ultra-brief-pulse stimuli)

| Dose level | Thymatron System IV | |
	Energy level[a] (%)	Charge (mcoul)
1[b]	5	25
2[c]	10[d]	50
3[e]	15	76
4	25	75
5	35	115
6	50	173
7	70	259
8	100	403

Note. amp = amperes; mcoul = millicoulombs; msec = milliseconds; sec = seconds; /sec = Hertz.
[a]Percent of maximum output charge.
[b]Start at dose level 1 for unilateral ECT in female patients.
[c]Start at dose level 2 for bilateral ECT in female patients or unilateral ECT in male patients.
[d]Steps constrained to units of 5%.
[e]Start at dose level 3 for bilateral ECT in male patients.

match stimulus intensity with seizure threshold, and it results in stimulation of many patients at doses much higher than seizure threshold.

In a more useful variation of this method, the *calculated-dose paradigm*, the initial dose selected is anticipated to be moderately suprathreshold for a typical patient with certain characteristics (e.g., age, gender, electrode placement) (Enns and Karvelas 1995). For example, some providers use a preselected-dose strategy based solely on the age of the patient, with dose (e.g., as a percentage of maximum output charge) set to the patient's age in decades. In this case, such a stimulus dose may be many times the seizure threshold for a substantial percentage of patients, particularly elderly ones. Some practitioners have recommended a modified preselected-dose strategy, using one-half the age of the patient as the starting stimulus dose (Petrides and Fink 1996), although this may compensate too much in the other direction, particularly with younger patients.

Using seizure threshold data obtained by the dose-titration method described in Tables 5–2 through 5–4 (modified from Coffey et al. 1995), one can ensure that the stimulus is at least moderately above the initial seizure threshold

Table 5–8.   Instructions for use of ultra-brief-pulse dose titration schedules shown in Tables 5–6 and 5–7

Threshold determination	1.	Start at level indicated by gender and electrode placement.
	2.	Increase level **one step** if restimulation is necessary.
	3.	If no adequate seizure has occurred after three stimulations at the first session (uncommon), jump **two levels** for the fourth stimulus.
	4.	If no adequate seizure has taken place after four stimulations at the first session (rare), abort the treatment session and go **one level** higher for initial stimulus at the second treatment session to continue titration.
Successive treatments	1.	After establishing the lowest threshold level needed to produce an adequate seizure, **increase four steps** for the next treatment with *unilateral* ECT and **two steps** with *bilateral* ECT.
	2.	Whenever any further increase in stimulus intensity is indicated because of a missed, abortive, or inadequate seizure (see Chapters 8 and 11), use **two-step increments** for both *unilateral* and *bilateral* ECT.

for the great majority of patients at the start of the ECT course by using a level 5 stimulus dose for females younger than age 60 years and a level 6 stimulus dose for everyone else. In Tables 5–9 and 5–10, this guideline is specifically spelled out for currently marketed U.S. ECT devices.

Because only about 40% of the variance in seizure threshold can be accounted for by factors such as age, gender, and electrode placement, even the calculated-dose technique still results in markedly suprathreshold stimuli for many patients. Also, as with any dosing technique, the variable rise in seizure threshold over the ECT course will often eventually require restimulation at a higher level in some patients.

EEG-Based Dosing

Certain EEG measures may reflect seizure adequacy and therefore could be useful in assisting practitioners in stimulus dosing (Mayur 2006) (see Chapters 8 and 11), although this point has been disputed (Perera et al. 2004). In this regard, the

Table 5–9. Pre-selected stimulus dosing techniques for MECTA devices (brief-pulse and ultra-brief-pulse stimuli)

Dose level	MECTA SR-1 and JR-1					MECTA SR-2 and JR-2		MECTA SpECTrum 4000Q/5000Q					MECTA SpECTrum 4000M/5000M	
	PW (msec)	F (/sec)	D (sec)	I (amp)	Charge (mcoul)	Energy level[a]	Charge (mcoul)	PW (msec)	F (/sec)	D (sec)	I (amp)	Charge (mcoul)	Stimulus level[a] (%)	Charge (mcoul)
5[b]	1.0	60	2.0	0.8	192	3.5	202	1.0	60	2.0	0.8	192	35	202
6[c]	1.0	90	2.0	0.8	288	5.0	288	1.0	60	3.0	0.8	288	50	288
7	1.4	90	2.0	0.8	403	7.0	403	1.0	60	4.5	0.8	432	70	403
8	2.0	90	2.0	0.8	576	10.0	576	1.0	60	6.0	0.8	576	100	576

Note. amp=amperes; mcoul=millicoulombs; msec=milliseconds; sec=seconds; /sec=Hertz.
[a]Percent of maximum output charge.
[b]Females younger than 60 years.
[c]All others.

Table 5–10. Pre-selected stimulus dosing techniques for Somatics Thymatron devices (brief-pulse and ultra-brief-pulse stimuli)

Dose level	Thymatron DGx		Thymatron System IV	
	Energy level[a]	Charge (mcoul)	Energy level[a]	Charge (mcoul)
5[b]	35	202	35	202
6[c]	50	288	50	288
7	70	403	70	403
8	100	576	100	576

Note. amp = amperes; mcoul = millicoulombs; msec = milliseconds; sec = seconds; /sec = Hertz.
[a]Percent of maximum output charge.
[b]Females younger than 60 years.
[c]All others.

MECTA spECTrum 5000 series ECT devices (http://mectacorp.com) offer an option that provides an automated estimate of the likelihood that a given ECT treatment is therapeutically potent (Krystal and Weiner 1994, Krystal et al. 1998, 2000). This estimate is based on how much certain EEG characteristics of the induced seizure differ from those produced by barely suprathreshold (and thereby therapeutically ineffective) unilateral ECT. This option also offers, for unilateral ECT, an automated estimate of the extent to which the stimulus that elicited the seizure exceeded seizure threshold. This latter feature would theoretically provide an ongoing means throughout the ECT course of assessing when a unilateral ECT stimulus comes too close to the seizure threshold and should be increased. The Somatics Thymatron System IV device (http://www.thymatron.com) also contains seizure quality features related to factors such as postictal EEG suppression, EEG seizure amplitude and coherence, and EEG seizure spectral content that could also theoretically be used for such purposes (Azuma et al. 2007).

Comparison of Dosing Methods

Each of these methods of stimulus dosing has both advantages and disadvantages. The dose-titration method is likely to result in a subconvulsive dose at the first treatment, necessitating restimulation (although our own experience over many years indicates that the median number of such restimulations at the first treatment is one). One advantage of this method is that the approximate seizure threshold at the time of the first treatment is determined, so that a moderate suprathreshold dose can be easily calculated. This is analogous to a pharmacological blood level in the sense that it offers a way to match the stimulus to a measurable criterion that is tied to clinical outcome. However, the variable rise in seizure threshold over the treatment course may diminish the usefulness of the initial dose determination in some patients.

With the preselected-dose method, only a very rough estimate of stimulus intensity can be made, even when considering factors such as age, gender, and electrode placement. The resulting stimuli may be grossly suprathreshold for some patients but subconvulsive or marginally suprathreshold for others. If a relatively high preselected dose is used, the clinician is less likely to administer a subconvulsive or marginally suprathreshold dose. Although the result may be more rapid or effective treatment (McCall et al. 1995), cognitive disturbances may be accentuated.

The EEG-based dosing technique, although promising, has not been sufficiently tested (at the time of writing) to be used on its own. However, the technique could well serve as an adjunct to either of the other dosing techniques, in the sense of providing some additional information to help guide the decision as to whether and when the stimulus dose should be increased over the treatment course.

We currently recommend the dose-titration technique as offering the most proven advantages. The reader should be aware, however, that the area of stimulus dosing remains under active study and that future findings may suggest an alternative methodology.

Electrode Placement

During the past decade, much discussion has occurred among practicing psychiatrists about which stimulus electrode placement to use for a given patient. There are two primary options, shown in Figure 5–2: bilateral placement and right unilateral placement. Other electrode placements, including bifrontal placement have also been proposed.

Bilateral and Right Unilateral Electrode Placement

ECT was originally delivered with bilateral placement, high stimulus dosing, and sine wave stimulus waveform. Each of these parameters has been associ-

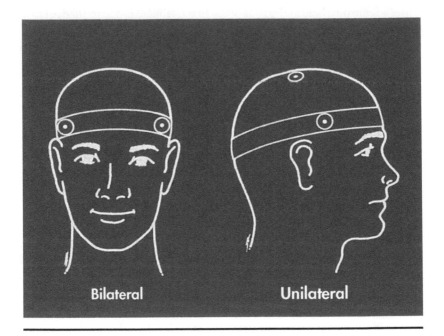

Figure 5–2.   Bilateral and right unilateral ECT electrode placement.

ated with increased cognitive side effects. As discussed in the preceding sections, moderately suprathreshold stimulus dosing and brief pulse stimulus were developed to optimize therapeutic potency and decrease adverse effects. Similarly, right unilateral electrode placement has also resulted in decreasing the cognitive side effects (Squire and Slater 1978; Strömgren et al. 1976). This decrease may be due in part to the relative sparing of nondominant mesial temporal lobe structures by both the stimulus current path and the induced seizure. The most commonly used unilateral placement is the d'Elia placement (d'Elia 1970), as demonstrated in Figure 5–2, although a variety of other unilateral placements have been proposed.

The controversy surrounding the choice in ECT of right unilateral versus bilateral electrode placement has been generated by mixed findings about efficacy, speed of action, and amount of cognitive side effects. Comparing studies is difficult, because results are confounded by differing stimulus intensities, lengths of treatments, patient diagnoses, outcome variables, and even specific choice of unilateral electrode placement. Despite this fact, the following statements appear to be supported by the majority of clinical research and experience:

1. Either technique is generally effective in the treatment of depression. However, some data suggest that specific subgroups, especially patients with mania, may not respond as thoroughly to unilateral treatments (Mukherjee et al. 1994).
2. In some studies, patients reportedly responded faster to bilateral placement, requiring fewer treatments for a course of ECT (Sackeim et al. 2000).
3. Some depressed patients who did not respond to right unilateral placement in ECT experienced significant clinical improvement after they were switched from unilateral to bilateral placement (Abrams et al. 1983).
4. Stimulus intensity just above seizure threshold markedly reduces the efficacy of unilateral ECT. This effect may be present to a lesser degree in bilateral ECT (Sackeim et al. 1993), particularly with ultra-brief-pulse stimuli.
5. Bilateral ECT results in greater acute cognitive side effects than does nondominant unilateral ECT. This difference is most apparent in tests assessing or requiring verbal function (Squire and Slater 1978). Also, although most memory functions appear to be restored in most patients 6 months after ECT, persisting memory complaints are more common in patients who receive bilateral ECT.

Because of the cognitive advantages of nondominant unilateral electrode placement over bilateral electrode placement, a reasonable approach is to routinely use nondominant unilateral ECT in patients who are more susceptible to profound confusional states. These patients may include those who are elderly, who have dementia, or who have developed significant confusion during prior courses of ECT. Unilateral ECT is also preferable for individuals who are highly concerned about the effects of ECT on memory functioning. Bilateral ECT is generally preferable for patients in whom a rapid response is clinically required (e.g., the actively suicidal patient or the catatonic patient who refuses to eat), as well as for those who have preferentially responded to bilateral ECT in the past or who indicate a preference for this modality.

A variation used by many clinicians is to begin with unilateral ECT and then switch to bilateral ECT if little or no therapeutic improvement is noted after six treatments. As with any major change regarding the ECT procedure, the clinician needs to discuss such changes with the consenter.

Determination of Cerebral Dominance

In individuals who are right motor dominant, the nondominant side of the brain with respect to speech functions is almost always the right side. With individuals who are left motor dominant, the situation is less clear (Pratt et al. 1971). In such cases, one may estimate dominance by use of a cognitive assessment technique carried out at the second and third ECT treatments. This technique involves giving a series of verbal recall tasks (e.g., "What are the names of these three objects?") as the patient awakens after each of the second and third ECT treatments. Right-side electrode placement is used for the first treatment, because that treatment involves dose titration to estimate seizure threshold. The second and third treatments are then given in either a right-left or a left-right sequence. To avoid confounding the data, the practitioner must use different objects for memory testing after each treatment. The nondominant hemisphere can then be assumed to be the side associated with the highest score on the verbal recall tasks. If scores from treatments 2 and 3 are equal, mixed dominance is implied, and either right or left unilateral ECT can be used (although right unilateral electrode placement is usually chosen because of convenience).

Bifrontal Electrode Placement

Several other ECT electrode placement strategies have been proposed, none of which has been studied with the depth of bilateral and right unilateral ECT. Of these alternatives, the most studied and most frequently used is bifrontal ECT. Bifrontal electrode placement has been proposed as a means to maintain the efficacy of traditional bilateral electrode placement while diminishing the level of memory impairment (possibly due to lessened seizure intensity in mesial temporal brain areas).

Data supporting the efficacy of bifrontal ECT have been reported in the treatment of both major depressive episodes (Eschweiler et al. 2007) and acute mania (Hiremani et al. 2008). However, the efficacy of bifrontal ECT compared with other electrode placements remains controversial (Bakewell et al. 2004; Heikman et al. 2002). These studies have supported a cognitive advantage for bifrontal over bilateral ECT, although such an advantage is unlikely with respect to right unilateral electrode placement.

Other Electrode Placements

Modified bilateral or right unilateral ECT may be indicated in cases of skull defects from head trauma or surgery. As noted in Chapter 4, placing electrodes over skull defects may substantially increase the amount of stimulus charge entering brain tissue. In patients with skull defects, physicians should avoid placing stimulus electrodes directly over the defects while closely approximating the routinely used electrode placement of choice for that patient. Neuroimaging studies, such as computed tomographic (CT) scan with "bone windows," may help in confirmation of actual skull defects rather than approximation of such defects by visual inspection or reliance on surgical scars.

References

Abrams R: Electroconvulsive Therapy, 4th Edition. New York, Oxford University Press, 2002

Abrams R, Taylor MA, Faber R, et al: Bilateral versus unilateral electroconvulsive therapy: efficacy in melancholia. Am J Psychiatry 140:463–465, 1983

American Psychiatric Association: The Practice of Electroconvulsive Therapy: Recommendations for Treatment, Training, and Privileging (A Task Force Report of the American Psychiatric Association), 2nd Edition. Washington, DC, American Psychiatric Publishing, 2001

Azuma H, Fujita A, Sato K, et al: Postictal suppression correlates with therapeutic efficacy for depression in bilateral sine and pulse wave electroconvulsive therapy. Psychiatry Clin Neurosci 61:168–173, 2007

Bakewell CJ, Russo J, Tanner C, et al: Comparison of clinical efficacy and side effects for bitemporal and bifrontal electrode placement in electroconvulsive therapy. J ECT 20:145–153, 2004

Coffey CE, Lucke J, Weiner RD, et al: Seizure threshold in electroconvulsive therapy, I: initial seizure threshold. Biol Psychiatry 37:713–720, 1995

d'Elia G: Unilateral electroconvulsive therapy. Acta Psychiatr Scand 215(suppl):1–98, 1970

Enns M, Karvelas L: Electrical dose titration for electroconvulsive therapy: a comparison with dose prediction methods. Convuls Ther 11:86–93, 1995

Eschweiler GW, Vonthein R, Bode R, et al: Clinical efficacy and cognitive side effects of bifrontal versus right unilateral electroconvulsive therapy (ECT): a short-term randomised controlled trial in pharmaco-resistant major depression. J Affect Disord 101:149–157, 2007

Frey R, Heiden A, Scharfetter J, et al: Inverse relation between stimulus intensity and seizure duration: implications for ECT procedure. J ECT 17:102–108, 2001

Heikman P, Kalska H, Katila H, et al: Right unilateral and bifrontal electroconvulsive therapy in the treatment of depression: a preliminary study. J ECT 18:26–30, 2002

Hiremani RM, Thirthalli J, Tharayil BS, et al: Double-blind randomized controlled study comparing short-term efficacy of bifrontal and bitemporal electroconvulsive therapy in acute mania. Bipolar Disord 10:701–707, 2008

Krystal AD, Weiner RD: ECT seizure therapeutic adequacy. Convuls Ther 10:153–164, 1994

Krystal AD, Coffey CE, Weiner RD, et al: Changes in seizure threshold over the course of electroconvulsive therapy affect therapeutic response and are detected by ictal EEG ratings. J Neuropsychiatry Clin Neurosci 10:178–186, 1998

Krystal AD, Weiner RD, Lindahl V, et al: The development and retrospective testing of an electroencephalographic seizure quality-based stimulus dosing paradigm with ECT. J ECT 16:338–349, 2000

Mayur P: Ictal electroencephalographic characteristics during electroconvulsive therapy: a review of determination and clinical relevance. J ECT 22:213–217, 2006

McCall WV, Farah BA, Reboussin D, et al: Comparison of the efficacy of titrated, moderate-dose and fixed, high-dose right unilateral ECT in elderly patients. Am J Geriatr Psychiatry 3:317–324, 1995

McCall WV, Reboussen DM, Weiner RD, et al: Titrated moderately suprathreshold vs. fixed high-dose right unilateral electroconvulsive therapy. Arch Gen Psychiatry 57:438–444, 2000

Mukherjee S, Sackeim HA, Schnur DB: Electroconvulsive therapy of acute manic episodes: a review of 50 years' experience. Am J Psychiatry 151:169–176, 1994

Ottosson JO: Experimental studies of the mode of action of electroconvulsive therapy. Acta Psychiatr Scand 35 (suppl):1–141, 1960

Perera TD, Luber B, Nobler MS, et al: Seizure expression during electroconvulsive therapy: relationships with clinical outcome and cognitive side effects. Neuropsychopharmacology 29:813–825, 2004

Petrides G, Fink M: The "half-age" stimulation strategy for ECT dosing. Convuls Ther 12:138–146, 1996

Pratt RT, Warrington EK, Halliday AM: Unilateral ECT as a test for cerebral dominance, with a strategy for treating left-handers. Br J Psychiatry 119:79–83, 1971

Sackeim HA, Decina P, Kanzler M, et al: Effects of electrode placement on the efficacy of titrated, low-dose ECT. Am J Psychiatry 144:1449–1455, 1987

Sackeim HA, Devanand DP, Prudic J: Stimulus intensity, seizure threshold, and seizure duration: impact on the efficacy and safety of electroconvulsive therapy. Psychiatr Clin North Am 14:803–843, 1991

Sackeim HA, Prudic J, Devanand DP, et al: Effects of stimulus intensity and electrode placement on the efficacy and cognitive effects of electroconvulsive therapy. N Engl J Med 328:839–846, 1993

Sackeim HA, Prudic J, Devanand DP, et al: A prospective, randomized double-blind comparison of bilateral and right unilateral electroconvulsive therapy at different stimulus intensities. Arch Gen Psychiatry 57:425–434, 2000

Squire SR, Slater PC: Bilateral and unilateral ECT: effects on verbal and nonverbal memory. Am J Psychiatry 135:1316–1320, 1978

Strömgren LS, Crhristensen AL, Fromholt P: The effects of unilateral brief-interval ECT on memory. Acta Psychiatr Scand 54:336–346, 1976

6

Anesthetics and Other Medications

Mehul V. Mankad, M.D.

Richard D. Weiner, M.D., Ph.D.

During the early years of ECT, electricity was applied to patients without anesthesia or muscle relaxation. Beginning in the 1950s and 1960s, however, several types of medication were introduced to increase the safety and patient acceptability of ECT. These medications included anesthetics, muscle relaxants, anticholinergics, and sympatholytic agents. Along with oxygenation and other refinements in the ECT technique (see Chapter 5, "Clinical Applications"; Chapter 7, "Ictal Motor Response"; Chapter 8, "Ictal Electroencephalographic Response"; and Chapter 9, "Cardiovascular Response"), these medications have resulted in much safer and more therapeutic ECT practice (American Psychiatric Association 2001; Ding and White 2002; Saito 2005). A list of the most commonly used medications given at the time of ECT administration is provided in Table 6–1.

Anesthetic Agents

The goal of anesthesia during ECT is to induce in the patient a brief period of amnesia covering the period of the electrical stimulation and the action of the muscle-relaxing agent. However, the level of anesthesia should not be so deep as to overly suppress the seizure activity, because that activity is the aim of the treatment.

The standard anesthetics used for ECT are barbiturates, of which methohexital (Brevital) is the most commonly used, followed by thiopental (Pentothal) (see Table 6–1 for typical doses). Methohexital has the advantages of rapid action, low cardiac toxicity, and a low incidence of postanesthesia confusion (Mokriski et al. 1992). In a recent systematic review, methohexital was shown to be superior to other anesthetics with regard to motor seizure duration (Hooten and Rasmussen 2008).

Because all barbiturates raise the seizure threshold and prolong the apneic period, titrating the dose of anesthetic is important. The recommended dose of methohexital is 0.75–1.0 mg/kg of body weight, given intravenously as a single bolus. This initial dose may be decreased if the patient is elderly or obese. Subsequent doses are adjusted according to the patient's previous response. The adequacy of anesthesia administered can generally be assessed by observing the patient for the presence of movements or unexplained autonomic activation (e.g., tachycardia) just before the stimulus. If a patient has not been adequately anesthetized, a small additional intravenous dose of anesthetic agent (e.g., 10–30 mg of methohexital) should be given immediately.

Propofol (Diprivan) is a newer nonbarbiturate agent that is less cardiotoxic than methohexital and also has a shorter half-life of action. Although it has been used successfully as the sole anesthetic in ECT, propofol is not recommended for routine ECT anesthesia because it substantially shortens seizure duration (and likely increases seizure threshold) compared with methohexital (Geretsegger et al. 2007; Walder et al. 2001), although the clinical significance of this effect has been questioned (Malsch et al. 1994). Recent reports indicate that the combination of propofol and an intravenous opiate such as remifentanil (Ultiva), alfentanil (Alfenta), or fentanyl (Fentora) may decrease the total amount of propofol required for anesthesia, thereby increasing seizure length and improving postictal suppression (Porter et al. 2008). Similar findings have been reported with such agents used in combination with other anesthetic medications used during ECT.

Table 6–1. Names and doses of medications commonly used during ECT

Medication	Dose
Anesthetic agents	
etomidate (Amidate)	0.2–0.6 mg/kg iv
ketamine (Ketalar)	1.5–2.0 mg/kg iv
methohexital (Brevital)	0.75–1.0 mg/kg iv
propofol (Diprivan)	1.0–1.5 mg/kg iv
thiopental (Pentothal)	2–4 mg/kg iv
Anticholinergic agents	
atropine (Atropine)	0.4–1.0 mg iv or 0.3–0.6 mg im
glycopyrrolate (Robinul)	0.2–0.4 mg iv, im, or sc
Benzodiazepine antagonist	
flumazenil (Romazicon)	0.5–1.0 mg iv
Muscle relaxants	
atracurium (Tracrium)	0.4–0.5 mg/kg iv
cisatracurium (Nimbex)	0.2 mg/kg iv
rocuronium (Zemuron)	0.6–1.3 mg/kg iv
succinylcholine (Anectine)	0.5–1.25 mg/kg iv
Postictal sedatives	
diazepam (Valium)	2.5–10 mg iv
haloperidol (Haldol)	2–10 mg iv
lorazepam (Ativan)	1–4 mg iv
midazolam (Versed)	0.5–2.0 mg iv
Sympatholytic agents	
esmolol (Brevibloc)	1 mg/kg iv (may also be used as an infusion)
labetalol (Trandate, Normodyne)	5–30 mg iv
nifedipine (e.g., Adalat)	10 mg sl
nitroglycerin (e.g., Nitrostat)	0.2–0.4 mg iv or sl (also patch and paste)

Note. im=intramuscularly; iv=intravenously; sc=subcutaneously; sl=sublingually.

Ketamine (Ketalar), another nonbarbiturate anesthetic agent, may be indicated when the maximum stimulus output of the ECT device has already been reached without a satisfactory ictal response. Although ketamine does not appear to elevate seizure threshold, it is slightly more cardiotoxic than bar-

biturates and also produces transient emergence psychosis in a minority of patients. For these reasons, it is not used as the routine anesthetic of choice.

The acceptance of etomidate (Amidate) as an anesthetic agent in ECT is
increasing. Etomidate has a favorable profile with regard to its low anticonvulsant effect, rapidity of induction and emergence, and limited adverse effect
profile. In head-to-head comparison, etomidate has shown marginal benefit
over propofol with regard to seizure length, amount of electrical charge necessary for adequate treatment, and total number of treatments during an index
course of ECT (Eranti et al. 2008; Patel et al. 2006). Widespread adoption of
etomidate is unlikely due to concern about acute adrenal insufficiency (a crit-
ical care emergency) after as little as a single induction dose of the drug
(Lundy et al. 2007).

Limited data exist for the use of inhalational anesthetics in ECT. Sevoflurane (Ultane) has been used safely as the primary anesthetic in some studies
(K. G. Rasmussen et al. 2007).

Muscle Relaxants

The use of muscle relaxants with ECT has improved airway management and almost completely eliminated musculoskeletal trauma as a complication of ECT.
Before these agents were used, fractures were a common complication in convulsive therapy (although they generally presented as asymptomatic spinal
compression fractures).

The goal of a muscle relaxant in ECT is to decrease the intensity of ictal
motor movements. Complete paralysis is neither necessary nor desirable in most
cases, because it may be associated with prolonged apnea. Exceptions to this
rule involve patients for whom even mild motor manifestations should be
avoided, such as some individuals with severe osteoporosis or those with fragile or unstable musculoskeletal disease.

The adequacy of muscle relaxation should be checked before stimulation.
Adequate relaxation can be confirmed by testing for a diminution of deep
tendon reflexes, loss of withdrawal (e.g., plantar) reflexes, and decreased muscle tone. Particularly in cases for which achievement of complete muscular
relaxation is essential, a peripheral nerve stimulator may be used. The stimulator is set to provide intermittent electrical pulses to a peripheral nerve (usually the posterior tibial nerve at the ankle or the median nerve at the wrist) at

a rate of one or two per second and at an intensity sufficient to produce a muscle twitch in response to each pulse. Typically, maximal relaxation is seen when the resultant muscle contraction (twitch) has stopped, although in practice this technique is not always reliable. Because peripheral nerve stimulation is uncomfortable, its use should be initiated only when the patient is anesthetized.

Succinylcholine (Anectine) is the preferred relaxant agent. It is administered intravenously by either bolus or drip. The usual dose is 0.75–1.25 mg/kg of body weight. Succinylcholine is a depolarizing agent; therefore, in most patients, fasciculations (twitches of muscle groups innervated by single motor neurons) will be seen beginning in the upper body and progressing distally. Maximal relaxation has been achieved when the fasciculations have disappeared. The maximal effect of succinylcholine is usually achieved in 1–3 minutes postinfusion, and paralysis disappears in most patients after 3–5 minutes.

Variations in succinylcholine metabolism are occasionally noted (Whittaker 1980). Patients with severe hepatic disease or nutritional deficiencies may metabolize succinylcholine more slowly than desirable. More commonly, inborn errors of succinylcholine metabolism exist, usually on a heterozygous basis. Homozygous pseudocholinesterase deficiency, fortunately very rare, can be associated with extremely prolonged apnea with succinylcholine, whereas heterozygous individuals have varying levels of pseudocholinesterase activity. Individuals with genetic enzymatic deficiencies often report a personal or family history of prolonged apnea following exposure to muscle relaxants. If either of these conditions is suspected, a test for pseudocholinesterase activity may be performed. Routine testing is not recommended. For a patient who tests positive for the homozygous state, the preferred alternative is to use another relaxant agent (as discussed later in this section), or very low doses of succinylcholine (1–5 mg intravenously [iv]) may be considered. The situation is less severe for individuals with the heterozygous state, although the succinylcholine dose should still be reduced in proportion to the diminution in enzyme function.

Drug interactions with succinylcholine do exist. Its metabolism is slightly prolonged with lithium, digoxin, and some antibiotic agents (Marco and Randels 1979). However, except in the case of the long-acting anticholinesterase agents (used rarely as a topical antiglaucoma medication), such interactions are typically not of sufficient concern to require the use of an alternative relaxant. A similar margin of safety appears to be present when succinylcholine is used with nootropic anticholinesterase agents.

Another potential concern with succinylcholine is its tendency to produce a transient rise in serum potassium (because of its depolarizing effect on muscle fibers). Although this is not a problem in the great majority of patients, a potential for dangerous hyperkalemia exists in individuals with pre-existing significant hyperkalemia; severe, widespread muscular rigidity; or third-degree burns. A nondepolarizing relaxant should be used in such cases. In addition, some cases of rigid catatonia may result in hyperkalemia that must be considered when ECT is incorporated into the treatment plan (Hudcova and Schumann 2006). A final group of patients for whom succinylcholine should not be used are those who have had a personal or family history of malignant hyperthermia with prior anesthesia. However, a history of neuroleptic malignant syndrome, which presents with symptoms similar to those of malignant hyperthermia (although milder), does not appear to increase the risk of malignant hyperthermia, except in the case of active neuroleptic malignant syndrome with severe and widespread muscular rigidity (in which case a nondepolarizing relaxant should be used).

Rocuronium (Zemuron), atracurium (Tracrium), and cisatracurium (Nimbex) have been used as alternatives to succinylcholine. These nondepolarizing muscle relaxants have significantly longer half-lives than succinylcholine. Therefore, their use is usually associated with prolonged apnea, although this effect is minimized by reversal with physostigmine (combined with atropine to negate the systemic cholinergic effects of physostigmine). Because these are nondepolarizing agents, muscle fasciculations will not be seen, and a peripheral nerve stimulator is often used to help determine the amount of relaxation.

Some patients report generalized muscle pain after ECT. This side effect may be due to the intense fasciculations that follow the administration of succinylcholine, although this etiology has been questioned (K. G. Rasmussen et al. 2008). A minority of practitioners premedicate affected patients with nonparalytic doses of a nondepolarizing relaxant to prevent such symptoms. In these cases, the agent (e.g., atracurium 3.0–4.5 mg iv) is administered several minutes before the anesthetic agent and succinylcholine. Because nondepolarizing relaxants are competitive with succinylcholine, the dose of succinylcholine needs to be increased by 10%–25% to achieve the same degree of muscle relaxation.

Anticholinergic Agents

During ECT, vagal reflexes are induced on two separate occasions. The first occurs immediately following the electrical stimulus and may be associated with a transient bradycardia or asystole, usually not lasting more than 5–7 seconds (Kaufman 1994). The second may occur as the seizure ends, when a resulting transient bradycardia may be associated with atrial or ventricular ectopy. Premedication with a muscarinic anticholinergic agent may decrease the likelihood and severity of bradycardia or asystole due to vagal effects (P. Rasmussen et al. 2007).

Anticholinergic agents also diminish the risk of aspiration from excessive secretions. Many physicians do not routinely use them because of a lack of controlled trials to prove that these medications clearly diminish morbidity, and because their use may be associated with an increase in ictal tachycardia. However, according to Gitlin et al. (1993), some patient subgroups, notably those receiving sympathetic blocking agents, may be at increased risk unless anticholinergic premedication is used. In addition, missed, or absent, seizures are associated with an increased likelihood of poststimulus asystole, leading some practitioners also to add anticholinergic premedication at the first treatment when a dose-titration technique is used (see Chapter 5).

The most commonly used anticholinergic preparations are glycopyrrolate (Robinul) (0.2–0.4 mg iv, intramuscularly, or subcutaneously) and atropine (Atropine) (0.4–1.0 mg iv or 0.3–0.6 mg intramuscularly or subcutaneously). Most practitioners prefer glycopyrrolate, because atropine is a centrally acting anticholinergic that crosses the blood-brain barrier and could theoretically exacerbate postictal delirium, although objective evidence for this is not compelling (Calev et al. 1993). Alternatively, some studies have shown atropine to be more potent in its effects on cardiac rhythm, both in protecting against bradycardia and asystole and in producing tachycardia (K. G. Rasmussen et al. 1999).

Anticholinergic medications can be administered in two different ways: 1) intravenously 2–3 minutes before the anesthetic agent or 2) subcutaneously or intramuscularly 30 minutes before the anesthetic agent. Most practitioners believe that when anticholinergic agents are given subcutaneously or intramuscularly, the reduction of oropharyngeal secretions is maximized, thereby improving airway management and reducing the risk of aspiration, although some data have questioned this advantage for the subcutaneous or intramuscular route (Kramer et al.

1992). When these medications are given intravenously, the cardiac effects can be directly observed (increased heart rate), dry mouth before the treatment can be avoided, and the patient does not have to endure the discomfort of an injection. Whatever route of administration is used, the practitioner should remember that individuals vary in their responses to a specific dose and that the anticholinergic effects of any concurrent medications should be taken into account.

Sympatholytic Agents

During ECT, the sympathetic nervous system is activated, resulting in a transient surge in systolic pressure and heart rate. This effect can present a significant physiological challenge to patients with hypertension or ischemic heart disease. Short-acting beta-blockers are often used to diminish the risk. However, the practitioner must avoid iatrogenically inducing a hypotensive state postictally, thereby increasing patients' fall risk as well as compromising cardiac patients.

Labetalol (Trandate, Normodyne) is the most commonly used beta-blocker at present. It both selectively blocks α_1-adrenergic receptors and nonselectively blocks β_1- and β_2-adrenergic receptors (Stoudemire et al. 1990). It is usually given in an intravenous bolus 2 minutes before anesthesia induction. Efficacy can be monitored by measuring blood pressure at a 2-minute interval postinjection. The usual starting dose is 5–10 mg given intravenously. Although prolonged or severe hypotension has not been reported after ECT using labetalol (Wegliski 1993), patients should be kept at bed rest for at least 1–2 hours postictally, because the functional half-life of this medication is at least 1–3 hours.

Esmolol (Brevibloc) is an ultra–short-acting beta-blocker now frequently used by anesthesiologists. Its half-life is 9 minutes after injection, thus decreasing the likelihood of post-ECT hypotension. Unfortunately, use of either esmolol or the longer-acting propranolol (Inderal) may shorten seizure duration compared with use of labetalol (McCall et al. 1997; van den Broek et al. 1999). Therefore, the usual practice is to reserve the use of esmolol to control sustained hypertension in the postictal period.

Importantly, the effects of beta-blockers on reducing cardiac rate are greater than they are on lowering blood pressure. Despite the theoretical concern that asystole might be lengthened during the early ictal response in the presence of a sympatholytic agent, studies have not shown this effect (Dannon et al. 1998).

In patients with significant hypertension, some anesthesiologists use alternative agents with more potent antihypertensive effects, such as nifedipine (e.g., Adalat) or nicardipine (Cardene) (either alone or in combination with a sympatholytic agent [Figiel et al. 1993]), when a marked attenuation of ECT-related hypertension is indicated. Nifedipine is usually administered sublingually 10–20 minutes before ECT. Nitroglycerin (e.g., Nitrostat), which is sometimes indicated at the time of ECT in patients with preexisting cardiac ischemic states (given sublingually, intravenously, or by patch), can be helpful in providing both antihypertensive and antibradycardic effects (Parab et al. 1992). In extreme situations, potent rapidly acting antihypertensive medications, such as nitroprusside (Nitropress), have also been used.

Oxygenation

Before the introduction of modified ECT with muscle relaxation, oxygen was not routinely used. During the convulsion, many patients significantly desaturated and became profoundly cyanotic. Use of muscle relaxants has decreased the body's requirement for additional oxygen, because oxygen-consuming muscular activity is substantially reduced. Even with this protection, however, cerebral oxygen consumption increases almost 200% during the seizure (Posner et al. 1969). Therefore, the patient should be ventilated with 100% oxygen at a rate of 15–20 breaths per minute, beginning approximately 1 minute before the induction of anesthesia and continuing until the resumption of spontaneous breathing. Patients with ischemic cardiac disease should receive a longer period of preoxygenation. The practitioner should be aware that hyperventilation decreases carbon dioxide saturation and thereby diminishes the drive to breathe postictally, particularly for patients with chronic obstructive pulmonary disease. The use of noninvasive oximetry to monitor arterial oxygen saturation is now a standard practice that enhances the safety of ECT.

Postictal Sedatives

An estimated 10% of ECT patients develop an acute confusional state, observed as the anesthetic wears off. This state is self-limited and is marked by agitation, disorientation, repetitive stereotyped movements, and failure to

respond to commands. Benzodiazepines may be used intravenously to terminate the symptoms; in recurrent cases, they may be used for prophylaxis. Most
practitioners administer the benzodiazepine after the patient begins breathing
but before the patient has regained full consciousness. Midazolam (Versed) and
lorazepam (Ativan) are the two agents most commonly used, and diazepam
(Valium) less frequently. Because midazolam (0.5–2.0 mg iv) may be the
shorter-acting of the two, it is most commonly used.

An alternative to benzodiazepines in the management and prevention of
postictal delirium is haloperidol (Haldol), which, when administered intravenously (as opposed to any other route), offers a prompt, brief sedation with
little or no extrapyramidal effects. An initial dose of 2–5 mg iv may be administered, followed by repeated doses at 2- to 3-minute intervals until the desired
effect is obtained. Because the duration of effect is very brief, repeat administration may sometimes be necessary.

In rare cases, the duration of action of the muscle relaxant significantly
exceeds that of the anesthetic agent, in which case the patient begins awakening while still paralyzed. In the absence of movement, this phenomenon is
heralded by hemodynamic signs of sympathetic arousal (i.e., tachycardia and
hypertension). In such situations, an anesthetic state should be rapidly reat-
tained, either via a repeat administration of the anesthetic agent used pre-
ictally or by giving a benzodiazepine as described above. Use of the cuff
technique decreases the likelihood of this phenomenon (see Chapter 7).

Benzodiazepine Antagonists

An attempt should be made to decrease or discontinue oral benzodiazepines
before ECT to avoid their anticonvulsant effect on the induced seizures (see
Chapter 3, "Patient Referral and Evaluation"). However, in many patients, an
urgent need for ECT, the presence of intense anxiety levels, or a concern
about provoking withdrawal symptoms may preclude such a decrease or dis-
continuation. In others, substantial benzodiazepine blood levels may persist
for days or even weeks following the last dose. Some practitioners use the benzodiazepine antagonist flumazenil (Romazicon) to reverse the action of these
agents at the time of ECT (Krystal et al. 1998). An intravenous bolus (0.5 mg)
is administered immediately after anesthesia induction but prior to administration of the muscle relaxant. In addition, because flumazenil's duration of

action can be an hour or more, a prudent action may be to treat patients who are still on relatively high doses of oral benzodiazepines with postictally administered intravenous benzodiazepine (e.g., midazolam 1–2 mg).

The availability of flumazenil has prompted some practitioners to consider the use of benzodiazepines for the acute management of high levels of anxiety before ECT on the treatment day itself (Bailine et al. 1994). This practice, however, should be reserved for extreme cases only.

References

American Psychiatric Association: The Practice of Electroconvulsive Therapy: Recommendations for Treatment, Training, and Privileging (A Task Force Report of the American Psychiatric Association), 2nd Edition. Washington, DC, American Psychiatric Publishing, 2001

Bailine SH, Saferman A, Vital-Herne J, et al: Flumazenil reversal of benzodiazepine-induced sedation for a patient with severe pre-ECT anxiety. Convuls Ther 10:65–68, 1994

Calev A, Fink M, Petrides G, et al: Caffeine pretreatment enhances clinical efficacy and reduces cognitive effects of electroconvulsive therapy. Convuls Ther 9:95–100, 1993

Dannon PN, Iancu I, Hirschmann S, et al: Labetalol does not lengthen asystole during electroconvulsive therapy. J ECT 14:245–250, 1998

Ding Z, White PF: Anesthesia for electroconvulsive therapy. Anesth Analg 94:1351–1364, 2002

Eranti SV, Mogg AJ, Pluck GC, et al: Methohexitone, propofol, and etomidate in electroconvulsive therapy for depression: a naturalistic comparison study. J Affect Disord 2008 Apr 23 [Epub ahead of print]

Figiel GS, DeLeo B, Zorumski CF, et al: Combined use of labetalol and nifedipine in controlling the cardiovascular response from ECT. J Geriatr Psychiatry Neurol 6:20–24, 1993

Geretsegger C, Nickel M, Judendorfer B, et al: Propofol and methohexital as anesthetic agents for electroconvulsive therapy: a randomized double-blind comparison of electroconvulsive therapy seizure quality, therapeutic efficacy, and cognitive performance. J ECT 23:239–243, 2007

Gitlin MC, Jahr JS, Margolis MA, et al: Is mivacurium chloride effective in electroconvulsive therapy? A report of four cases, including a patient with myasthenia gravis. Anesth Analg 77:392–394, 1993

Hooten WM, Rasmussen KG: Effects of general anesthetics in adults receiving electroconvulsive therapy: a systematic review. J ECT 24:208–223, 2008

Hudcova J, Schumann R: Electroconvulsive therapy complicated by life-threatening hyperkalemia in a catatonic patient. Gen Hosp Psychiatry 28:440–442, 2006

Kaufman KR: Asystole with electroconvulsive therapy. J Intern Med 235:275–277, 1994

Kramer BA, Afrasiabi A, Pollock VE: Intravenous versus intramuscular atropine in ECT. Am J Psychiatry 149:1258–1260, 1992

Krystal AD, Watts BV, Weiner RD, et al: The use of flumazenil in the anxious and benzodiazepine-dependent ECT patient. J ECT 14:5–14, 1998

Lundy JB, Slane ML, Frizzi JD: Acute adrenal insufficiency after a single dose of etomidate. J Intensive Care Med 22:111–117, 2007

Malsch E, Gratz I, Mani S, et al: Efficacy of electroconvulsive therapy after propofol and methohexital anesthesia. Convuls Ther 10:212–219, 1994

Marco LA, Randels PM: Succinylcholine drug interactions during electroconvulsive therapy. Biol Psychiatry 14:433–445, 1979

McCall WV, Zvara D, Brooker R, et al: Effect of esmolol pretreatment on EEG seizure morphology in RUL ECT. Convuls Ther 13:175–180, 1997

Mokriski BK, Nagle SE, Papuchis GC, et al: Electroconvulsive therapy-induced cardiac arrhythmias during anesthesia with methohexital, thiamylal, or thiopental sodium. J Clin Anesth 4:208–212, 1992

Parab AL, Chaudari LS, Apte J: Use of nitroglycerin ointment to prevent hypertensive response during electroconvulsive therapy: a study of 50 cases. J Postgrad Med 38:55–57, 1992

Patel AS, Gorst-Unsworth C, Venn RM, et al: Anesthesia and electroconvulsive therapy: a retrospective study comparing etomidate and propofol. J ECT 22:179–183, 2006

Porter R, Booth D, Gray H, et al: Effects of the addition of remifentanil to propofol anesthesia on seizure length and postictal suppression index in electroconvulsive therapy. J ECT 24:203–207, 2008

Posner JB, Plum F, Van Poznak A: Cerebral metabolism during electrically induced seizures in man. Arch Neurol 20:388–395, 1969

Rasmussen KG, Jarvis MR, Zormuski CF, et al: Low-dose atropine in electroconvulsive therapy. J ECT 15:213–221, 1999

Rasmussen KG, Laurila DR, Brady BM, et al: Anesthesia outcomes in a randomized double-blind trial of sevoflurane and thiopental for induction of general anesthesia in electroconvulsive therapy. J ECT 23:236–238, 2007

Rasmussen KG, Petersen KN, Sticka JL, et al: Correlates of myalgia in electroconvulsive therapy. J ECT 24:84–87, 2008

Rasmussen P, Andersson JE, Koch P, et al: Glycopyrrolate prevents extreme bradycardia and cerebral deoxygenation during electroconvulsive therapy. J ECT 23:147–152, 2007

Saito S: Anesthesia management for electroconvulsive therapy: hemodynamic and respiratory management. J Anesth 19:142–149, 2005

Stoudemire A, Knos G, Gladson M, et al: Labetalol in the control of cardiovascular responses to electroconvulsive therapy in high-risk depressed medical patients. J Clin Psychiatry 51:508–512, 1990

van den Broek WW, Leentjens AF, Mulder PG, et al: Low-dose esmolol reduces seizure duration during electroconvulsive therapy: a double-blind, placebo-controlled study. Br J Anaesth 83:271–274, 1999

Walder B, Seeck M, Tramer MR: Propofol versus methohexital for electroconvulsive therapy: a meta-analysis. J Neurosurg Anesthesiol 13:93–98, 2001

Wegliski M: New anesthetic agents used in electroconvulsive therapy. Psychiatr Ann 23:23–26, 1993

Whittaker M: Plasma cholinesterase variants and the anaesthetist. Anaesthetist 35:174–197, 1980

PART 3

Seizure Monitoring

7

Ictal Motor Response

Andrew D. Krystal, M.D., M.S.

The purpose of the electrical stimulus in ECT is to induce a generalized grand mal type of seizure. The seizure produced is not an all-or-nothing phenomenon. As mentioned in Chapter 5, "Clinical Applications," and Chapter 6, "Anesthetics and Other Medications," various factors can influence seizure threshold, the physiological effects of the seizure, the associated cognitive side effects, and the seizure's therapeutic efficacy. The physician administering ECT must be able to determine whether a seizure has been elicited, assess the therapeutic adequacy of the induced seizure, determine the duration of the seizure, and respond appropriately when seizures are missed, inadequate, or prolonged.

Various types of data have to be monitored simultaneously during an ECT treatment. These include the patient's motor response, blood pressure, pulse rate, electroencephalographic (EEG) and (in some cases) electromyographic (EMG) data, and oxygen saturation. Adequately monitoring all of these things can be overwhelming to the novice. However, understanding the basic principles involved and the range of anticipated findings makes this situation considerably less difficult. In the next three chapters, we review the principles underlying the various modalities monitored during ECT and discuss how to interpret the clinical implications of the findings. This chapter focuses on monitoring the patient's motor activity. Ictal EEG activity is the subject of Chapter 8, "Ictal Electroencephalographic Response," and the cardiovascular response to ECT is discussed in Chapter 9, "Cardiovascular Response."

Motor Seizure Monitoring

Generalized grand mal types of seizures can be monitored both by observing the ictal motor response (convulsion) and by monitoring ictal EEG activity (the electrophysiological activity of the brain occurring during the seizure). Ictal EEG monitoring has been recommended for routine use for several reasons: 1) it reflects the action of the organ that is actually generating the seizure (i.e., the brain); 2) EEG seizure activity is typically 10–20 seconds longer (and occasionally much longer) than motor activity; 3) the motor response may not always be observable, or in some cases no motor response may occur during the seizure; and 4) prolonged seizures may be detectable only by EEG (American Psychiatric Association 2001; Weiner et al. 1991).

Monitoring motor activity is useful as well, however, because EEG monitoring may sometimes be unreliable, particularly in the presence of artifact. Evidence of seizure may be observed in the motor response before it is apparent in the EEG.

Ictal Motor Response

During the electrical stimulus itself, many muscle groups may contract, causing extension of the neck, flexion of the ankle, and clenching of the jaw. This response is not ictal but is due to the direct electrical effects of the stimulation. It can readily be distinguished from the seizure, because these contractions immediately disappear upon termination of the electrical stimulus and cannot be blocked with the use of a muscle relaxant, such as succinylcholine.

A gradual, sustained tonic contraction represents the first phase of the ictal motor response, and it usually occurs either immediately or within a few seconds after termination of the stimulus. Barely suprathreshold seizures may be associated with a delay of motor response of up to 10 seconds. Overall, the tonic phase of the ictal motor response may last from a few seconds to tens of seconds. Gradually, it evolves into the clonic phase, a period of rhythmic alterations in flexion and extension that decrease in frequency over time, then abruptly terminate. The clonic phase typically lasts longer than the tonic phase.

Factors Influencing the Motor Response

The intensity of convulsive motor activity is influenced by two factors: the dose of muscle relaxant (generally succinylcholine) and, to a lesser degree, the intensity of the electrical stimulus (Weiner et al. 1991). The dose of succinylcholine determines the level of muscular relaxation. A dose of 0.5–0.75 mg/kg often provides incomplete relaxation; thus, convulsive movements may be prominent. A routine dose of 1.0 mg/kg usually causes complete or nearly complete relaxation of the muscles, resulting in mild, or even absent, convulsive activity. Occasionally, larger doses may be needed, particularly in patients with orthopedic problems or in patients who have received premedication with nondepolarizing muscle relaxants (see Chapter 3, "Patient Referral and Evaluation," and Chapter 6, "Anesthetics and Other Medications").

Because muscle relaxants may block observable convulsive activity, the clinician may have difficulty determining whether an ictal motor response has started or when it is completed. Therefore, most physicians use a practice known as the *cuff technique* to allow the motor convulsion to be monitored. Just before the muscle relaxant is administered, a blood pressure cuff is placed on a distal extremity (wrist or ankle) and inflated well above the systolic pressure (about 200 mm Hg). This procedure prevents the flow of muscle relaxant distal to the cuff and enables unblocked muscles to manifest convulsive activity. The ankle is generally preferable to the wrist because it is a more stable joint and the cuff does not interfere with intravenous lines or blood pressure monitoring. The cuff pressure should be released as soon as a seizure has occurred to minimize the risks associated with a loss of vascular perfusion to the region distal to the cuff. Special care should be taken in patients who have 1) major musculoskeletal disease distal to the cuff (e.g., severe osteoporosis), 2) severe vascular insufficiency (e.g., decreased perfusion due to diabetes), or

3) sickle cell anemia and any other blood-clotting abnormalities that may precipitate local clotting. In severe examples of such conditions, the cuff technique should not be used.

Convulsive movements may also be present in areas other than the cuffed extremity, and they may not always end simultaneously in all locations (Weiner et al. 1991). Because of this variability, physicians sharing ECT administration duties at the same facility should adopt a standard convention as to what constitutes the end of the motor convulsion (American Psychiatric Association 2001). This convention may be based on 1) the cessation of movements in the cuffed extremity or 2) the longest-lasting motor activity observed in either the cuffed or the homologous extremity or anywhere in the body.

The second factor influencing the intensity of the ictal motor response is the intensity of the electrical stimulation. As noted in Chapter 5, the ictal motor response to stimuli barely above threshold may sometimes be attenuated or totally absent.

Electromyography

Another technique for monitoring ictal motor activity is to record the electrical activity produced by the muscles themselves—that is, EMG activity (Weiner et al. 1991). EMG activity provides a physiological index of motor activity that may be more sensitive than that obtained by the cuff technique, although EMG activity is also more likely to be affected by artifact. Although EMG activity has not traditionally been recorded during ECT, both the MECTA spECTrum 5000Q (http://www.mectacorp.com) and the Somatics Thymatron System IV (http://www.thymatron.com) ECT machines can be used to monitor EMG activity.

To record the EMG activity, a pair of recording electrodes, which can usually be the same as those used for EEG recording (see Chapter 8), are placed on the skin overlying muscles in any of a variety of sites. For use with ECT, however, they are typically located distal to the blood pressure cuff (on the cuffed extremity) to ensure a good EMG signal. The two leads are typically placed on the dorsum of the foot, approximately 3–4 inches apart (see Figure 7–1). In attaching the electrodes, attention must be given to good skin contact to minimize artifact. For this reason, good practice involves lightly abrading the underlying skin with a substance such as Omni Prep (D.O.

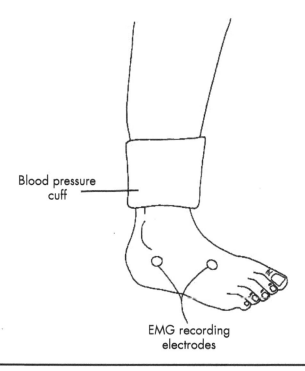

Blood pressure
cuff

EMG recording
electrodes

Figure 7–1. Electromyographic (EMG) electrode placement.

Weaver and Company) and wiping the area dry before applying the electrodes. Also, at least one of the recording electrodes should be placed directly over muscle tissue, because otherwise no EMG activity can be recorded.

Figure 7–2 demonstrates examples of an EMG recording made during the tonic (A) and clonic (B and C) portions of the seizure. The slow waves seen in the last EMG recording (C) reflect the presence of foot movement during the clonic phase. The Somatics Thymatron DGx device contains a feature that automatically detects the motor seizure end point on the basis of the EMG recording. An example of a typical EMG seizure end point is shown in Figure 7–3. In this case, the Thymatron device correctly estimated the motor end point at 45 seconds. Although EMG recording devices accurately show the seizure end point the majority of the time, the presence of artifact sometimes creates inaccuracies (Krystal and Weiner 1995).

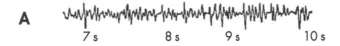

A
7 s   8 s   9 s   10 s

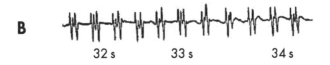

B
32 s   33 s   34 s

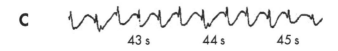

C
43 s   44 s   45 s

Figure 7–2.   Electromyographic (EMG) activity during the tonic (A) and clonic (B and C) portions of the seizure.

EMG activity was recorded from two electrodes located on the dorsum of the cuffed right foot.

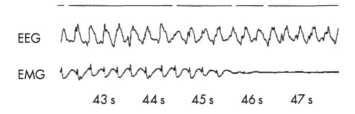

EEG

EMG
43 s   44 s   45 s   46 s   47 s

Figure 7–3.   Accurate Thymatron automatic detection of seizure end point.

EMG = electromyographic.

The dark line above the electroencephalographic (EEG) tracing denotes the device's determination that EEG seizure activity persists beyond termination of motor seizure activity.

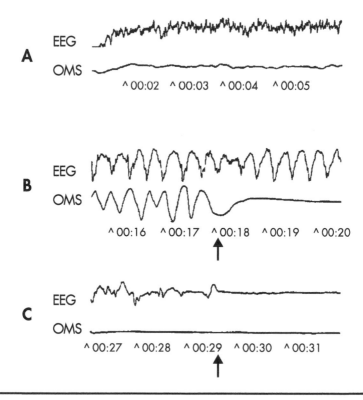

Figure 7–4. Ictal motor activity recorded using the optical motion sensor (OMS) technique.

(A) Seizure onset; (B) end of motor convulsion (arrow); and (C) end of electroencephalographic (EEG) seizure (arrow).

Photoplethysmography

Yet another means of automatically monitoring the motor response is represented by the optical motion sensor feature, which is optional with the MECTA spECTrum Q series devices (5000Q and 4000Q). A photoplethysmographic sensor is used to provide a signal reflecting the movements that occur during the clonic phase of the seizure. The sensor is strapped to a toe or finger distal to the blood pressure cuff used to prevent flow of succinylcholine to the foot or hand (as described above with the cuff technique); movements during the clonic phase are reflected as slow waves in the device's display panel and/or chart recorder output. When enough of a deflection is present, and artifacts are minimal, the termination of these slow waves provides an indication of when ictal motor activity has ceased (Figure 7–4B). In the absence of artifact, no optical motion sensor activity is observed during either the tonic portion of the seizure (Figure 7–4A) or the postictal phase (Figure 7–4C). However, artifacts can occur; potentially the most troublesome is pulse artifact, which can be minimized by keeping the cuff inflated until the ictal motor response is clearly over.

References

American Psychiatric Association: The Practice of Electroconvulsive Therapy: Recommendations for Treatment, Training, and Privileging (A Task Force Report of the American Psychiatric Association), 2nd Edition. Washington, DC, American Psychiatric Publishing, 2001

Krystal AD, Weiner RD: ECT seizure duration: reliability of manual and computer-automated determinations. Convuls Ther 11:158–169, 1995

Weiner RD, Coffey CE, Krystal AD: The monitoring and management of electrically induced seizures. Psychiatr Clin North Am 14:845–869, 1991

8

Ictal Electroencephalographic Response

Andrew D. Krystal, M.D., M.S.

Ictal Electroencephalographic Monitoring

When a seizure occurs during ECT, the activation of neurons produces a distinctive pattern of activity within the dendritic fields of large cortical pyramidal cells. When this activity becomes synchronous across many adjacent neurons, the resulting fluctuations in voltage can be detected at the scalp in the form of a signal known as the electroencephalogram (Weiner et al. 1991).

Electroencephalographic (EEG) signals are often characterized by their amplitude and frequency. *Amplitude* is an indicator of the size of the signal as reflected in the peak fluctuations in electrical voltage. At rest, EEG amplitudes range from 10 to 100 microvolts (μV). An example of typical EEG activity during the waking state in an adult is shown in Figure 8–1. In that example, the electroencephalogram has a maximum amplitude of around 50–60 μV. During a grand mal seizure, when many neurons have synchronous depolarizations, EEG

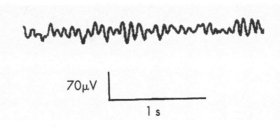

Figure 8–1.   Waking electroencephalogram.

s=second.

Maximum peak-to-peak amplitude is 50–60 µV. Dominant frequency is 12 Hz.

amplitudes can increase to 1,000 µV or more. After the seizure has concluded, this intense neuronal hyperactivity is followed by a profound inhibitory response, because of which postictal EEG amplitudes may decrease to as little as 1–10 µV.

EEG *frequency* refers to the number of cycles per second and is measured in hertz (Hz). Traditionally, the electroencephalogram is divided into four frequency bands: delta (0–4 Hz), theta (5–7 Hz), alpha (8–13 Hz), and beta (>13 Hz). EEG signals typically consist of the summation of many oscillating components at different frequencies. The largest component is referred to as the dominant frequency of the signal. The electroencephalogram in Figure 8–1 has a dominant frequency of 12 Hz. As shown in Figure 8–2, frequency differs across recording locations and states of consciousness. Low-voltage fast activity in the beta range predominates frontally in the waking state (Figure 8–2A). A strong alpha rhythm is typically seen posteriorly in the waking state, particularly when the eyes are closed (Figure 8–2B). Although theta and delta band rhythms (often called *slowing*) are usually abnormal in adults during the waking state, they normally occur during sleep, whether occurring naturally or induced by a general anesthetic (Figure 8–2C). However, an additional feature with barbiturate-induced sleep is fast activity in the beta range (Figure 8–2C).

Artifacts are aspects of the EEG signal that come from sources other than the electrical activity of the brain. These signals interfere with the ability to monitor brain electrical activity and most frequently derive from electrical equipment in the treatment room, eye movements, other body movements, muscle activity, and the heart (see Figure 8–9, later in chapter).

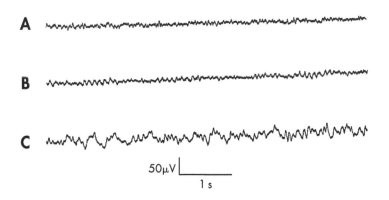

Figure 8–2.   Typical electroencephalographic activity during the waking state (A, B) and during anesthesia (C).

Electroencephalograms A and C were recorded frontally; electroencephalogram B was recorded occipitally. s=seconds.

Most U.S. ECT devices incorporate EEG monitoring capability with at least two-channel paper-output capability. (An option with the MECTA spECTrum Q series [http://www.mectacorp.com] and the Somatics Thymatron System IV [http://www.thymatron.com] devices allows up to four channels of EEG activity to be recorded.) Recording more channels decreases the likelihood that artifacts will make it impossible to monitor EEG activity in a given patient. However, this benefit must be weighed against 1) the extra time and complexity of recording more channels of data and 2) the fact that only in very rare instances are more than two channels needed for effective EEG monitoring.

Thymatron ECT devices additionally include an audible EEG monitor, which modulates an audible tone with the variation in ictal EEG activity and gives the practitioner a nonvisual reflection of EEG seizure activity (Swartz and Abrams 1986). The audible EEG monitor is generally used as a supplement to, rather than a replacement of, the paper recording, because the paper provides a permanent record of ictal events; this record can be particularly important in cases in which it is difficult to determine if a seizure has been elicited or the seizure end point (discussed later in "Determination of Seizure End Point") is unclear.

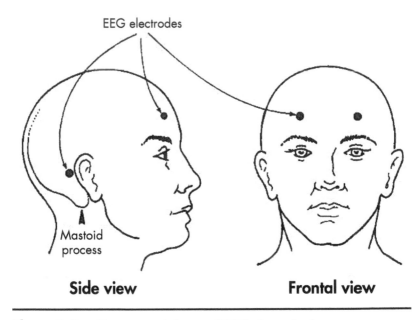

Figure 8–3.   Electroencephalogram (EEG) electrode placement.

EEG Electrode Placement

An EEG channel measures the difference in voltage over time (as variations in amplitude) between two scalp EEG recording electrode sites. Because of the desirability to know which cerebral hemisphere is generating the recorded activity, both recording electrodes in a given pair should be placed over the same cerebral hemisphere. When one- or two-channel EEG recording is used, prefrontal and mastoid locations (Figure 8–3) are preferred, for several reasons: 1) EEG amplitude during electrically induced seizures is often relatively high in frontal areas; 2) the mastoid location (just behind the ear) is a relatively inactive area electrophysiologically, thus making it a good reference for contrasting with the more active prefrontal area; and 3) both prefrontal and mastoid regions are relatively free of hair, making attachment of the electrodes easy.

Recording a single channel from electrodes placed in the right and left prefrontal areas is not recommended. Although convenient, this practice re-

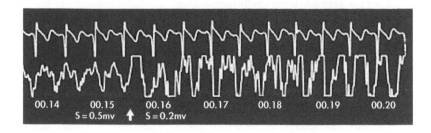

Figure 8–4. Electroencephalographic recording illustrating clipping of waveforms after the gain was increased at the arrow notation.

sults in EEG data that are harder to read. The reason is that the high-amplitude electrical activity that is often elicited with ECT seizures is manifested equally in these two regions, and by taking the difference between them, this activity is cancelled out and does not appear in the EEG signal.

Because the EEG signal is low in amplitude, contact between the electrode and scalp needs to be optimized. First, excess skin oil and debris should be removed from the recording electrode sites by mildly abrading the underlying scalp area with a rough gauze wetted with a solvent with abrasive properties (e.g., Omni Prep [D.O. Weaver and Company]). The solvent then should be wiped off and the area dried. Second, the recording electrodes should be well attached to the scalp. Self-adhesive pediatric electrocardiographic (ECG) recording pads are used by many practitioners.

Setting the Display and Printout Gain

The output gain is the ratio of the size of the signal displayed on a monitor or paper printout to the size of the recorded EEG signal. All ECT devices provide the capacity to adjust the output gain. The gain for all outputs should be set to make optimal use of the scale provided. If the gain is too low, the capacity to interpret the data is diminished. If the gain is too high, parts of the signal extend beyond the range displayed, creating the appearance that the tops of the waveforms are chopped off (see Figure 8–4). This so-called clipping also decreases the ability to interpret the data. The gain setting can be optimized through the following procedure:

1. Turn the gain up to the maximum setting.
2. If clipping of the electroencephalogram is observed, make certain it is not due to artifact (as discussed in "EEG Artifacts," later in this chapter). If not, turn the gain down a small amount.
3. Continue this process until the highest-amplitude nonartifact ictal EEG data observed just touch the top of the display or printout without clipping.
4. Use this same gain to monitor treatments for all subjects. (Marking the device to indicate the optimal setting is recommended if other people might change the setting.)

EEG interpretation is a pattern recognition skill, and altering the gain settings changes the pattern and can impede the capacity to interpret the data.

Prestimulus Electroencephalogram

The immediate prestimulus electroencephalogram is generally noticeably different from the patient's baseline waking electroencephalogram because of the effects of the anesthetic administered. However, the effects of the anesthetic on the electroencephalogram may be quite variable (see Figure 8–2C and Figure 8–11). The EEG effects depend on both the type of anesthetic used and the blood level of the agent.

An extremely helpful practice is to note or play out onto paper a brief period (at least 5–10 seconds) of immediate prestimulus EEG data (as close to the time of the stimulus as possible). This pretreatment strip is necessary to ensure that the EEG recording apparatus is functioning properly and that the signal is of acceptable quality (relatively free of artifacts). If the pretreatment electroencephalogram is not acceptable, steps should be taken to address the problem, such as making sure that the cables are plugged in properly, further cleaning of the scalp, or reattaching of the electrodes. The prestimulus electroencephalogram can also be useful for determining whether or not a seizure has been elicited, and occasionally it may help in determining the seizure end point.

During the period of electrical stimulation, EEG activity is blocked because of interference by the stimulus current. ECT devices generally begin recording only after the stimulus has been administered.

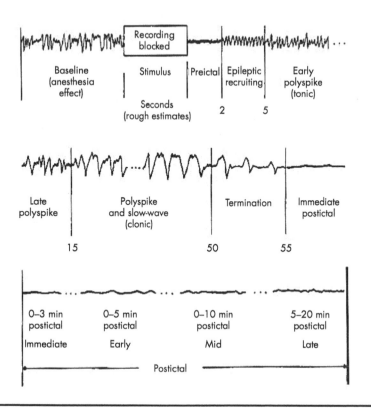

Figure 8–5. Schematic of various phases of a typical ECT seizure.

Source. Adapted from Weiner et al. 1991.

Ictal EEG Phases

Figure 8–5 illustrates typical ictal and postictal EEG phases that may be observed during the ECT treatment. The appearance of the electroencephalogram during ECT-induced seizures is quite variable. As shown in the figure, a characteristic evolution of EEG activity often occurs over the course of seizures. For the purposes of pedagogy, this continuous process has been broken down into a series of discrete stages that are often, but not always, present in the ictal electroencephalogram. Commonly, identifying one or more of these stages in the ictal electroencephalogram is impossible. The purpose of this section is to review the possible variations in ictal EEG morphology in greater depth.

Preictal Activity

After the electrical stimulus, a brief preictal period of relative suppression of EEG activity can occur, or low-amplitude fast activity can sometimes be seen.

Epileptic Recruiting Rhythm

The preictal activity may be followed by a brief period of very rhythmic activity of low to moderate amplitude in the alpha or beta range. This epileptic recruiting rhythm is believed to be associated with the synchronizing effects of thalamocortical projections during the early stages of seizure generalization.

Polyspike Activity

Often, the earliest phase of the seizure noted is that characterized by high-frequency activity with interspersed lower-frequency waveforms. This polyspike activity phase is concurrent with the tonic and early clonic components of the motor response and usually lasts approximately 10–15 seconds. It may be masked by electromyographic (EMG) artifact.

Polyspike and Slow-Wave Complexes

During the clonic phase of the ictal motor response, the polyspike activity evolves into repetitive polyspike and slow-wave complexes, which are synchronous with the clonic movements. During the beginning of the clonic motor phase, the frequency of these discharges is often 5 Hz or greater, although the frequency diminishes to as low as 1 Hz as the clonic phase progresses.

Termination Phase

Perhaps better referred to as the transition phase, the termination phase is marked by changes in EEG activity that accompany the transition from the ictal to the postictal state. This process is extremely variable. On some electroencephalograms, an abrupt transition occurs from classic polyspike and slow-wave activity to postictal activity (see Figures 8–5 and 8–6). On other electroencephalograms, one can see a continuous decrease in the frequency of

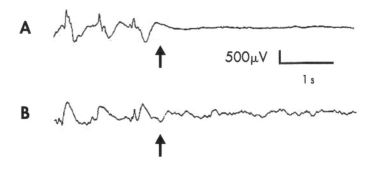

Figure 8–6. Determination of electroencephalographic (EEG) seizure end point.

s = second.

(A) Typical EEG seizure end point with abrupt end of seizure (at arrow), followed by flat postictal baselines. (B) Same as A, except that the postictal activity is not flat (arrow denotes seizure end point).

slow waves and/or slow-wave amplitude, multiple stepwise decreases in EEG amplitude (see Figure 8–7), or even brief periods (rarely up to 5 seconds) of apparent postictal suppression followed by resumption of ictal activity (see Figure 8–8).

Postictal Phase

The postictal phase begins at the point of EEG seizure termination (see Figure 8–5). The electroencephalogram may appear flat or nearly so. However, significantly higher amplitude may be seen if the degree of postictal suppression is relatively low; this is most likely to occur when the stimulus intensity is relatively close to the seizure threshold (Krystal and Weiner 1995; Krystal et al. 1993). In some cases, the degree of suppression is so minimal that the immediate prestimulus EEG pattern will reemerge at the end of the seizure. It is important to note that when the electroencephalogram appears to be flat, there is still ongoing EEG activity. The appearance of flatness is dependent on the display gain setting. With optimal gain settings, vigorous seizures typically lead to flat-appearing postictal EEG activity with the size of output displays most often used. Typically, the postictal electroencephalogram rises in both

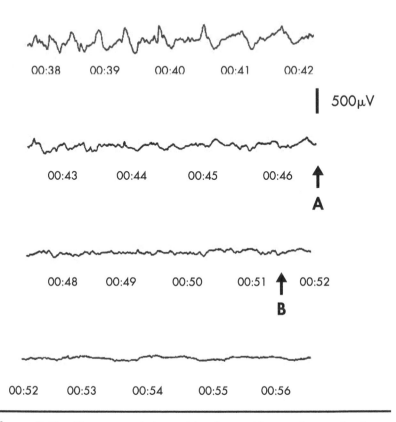

Figure 8–7. Electroencephalographic seizure with stepwise termination phase, eventually dissipating into a relatively flat postictal baseline. The seizure end point is at arrow B rather than arrow A.

amplitude and frequency over a period of minutes following the end of the seizure as it moves toward the preanesthetic baseline.

EEG Artifacts

To make the necessary clinical interpretations of EEG data (the determination of whether a seizure is present and, if so, where the seizure ends), the physician needs to be able to differentiate between electrical activity de-

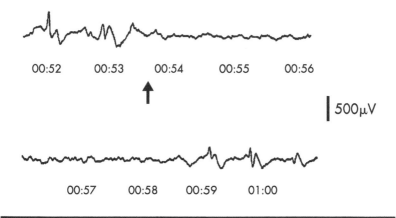

Figure 8–8. Electroencephalographic seizure that appears to end (at arrow) but resumes 5 seconds later.

riving from the brain and artifacts. The main types of artifacts encountered are muscle artifact, movement artifact, electrode contact artifact, and ECG artifact (see Figure 8–9).

Muscle Artifact

Electromyography reflects electrical potentials generated by muscle tissue, which typically appear as very-high-frequency (>30 Hz) components of the signal. They make the signal look dark or spiky as in Figure 8–9A. As shown in this figure, ictal muscle artifact can sometimes be so great as to obscure the ictal EEG patterns. The clinician should keep in mind that this activity coincides with motor activity during the seizure. In the tonic phase, ictal muscle artifact is generated by continuous muscular contraction and has a constant appearance in the signal. As the seizure evolves into the clonic phase, the EMG artifact takes on the pseudoperiodic quality of the convulsive movements. The EMG activity also disappears when the motor activity ceases. Although the motor seizure end point may sometimes be concurrent with the end of the EEG seizure, it typically occurs earlier, with a median time difference of about 15 seconds between the two measures, although the EEG activity may at times persist several minutes after the end of motor activity (Liston et al. 1988). The motor end point is not generally associated with any specific EEG correlates.

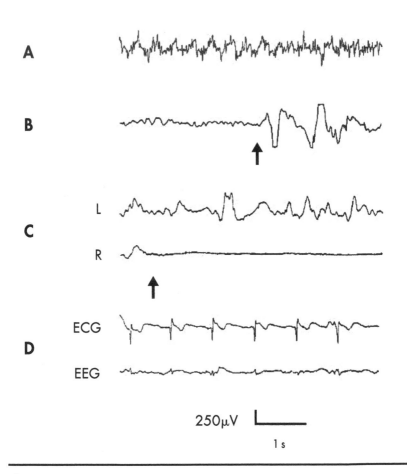

Figure 8–9.   Artifacts observed in ictal electroencephalographic (EEG) recording.

s = second.

(A) Continual electromyographic activity during the polyspike and slow-wave phase of a seizure. (B) Movement artifact, beginning at the arrow. (C) Artifact from a loose recording electrode on the left side (L). The end of the EEG seizure is shown by the arrow on the intact right-side recording (R). (D) Electrocardiographic (ECG) artifact in the EEG channel during the postictal state.

Movement Artifact

Another type of commonly encountered EEG artifact is movement artifact. This artifact is associated with deflections (gross shifts in the signal baseline) in the electroencephalogram, which are usually (but not always) different in shape from the ongoing activity just prior to the movement. An example of movement artifact is shown in Figure 8–9B, beginning at the arrow; in this case, the artifact was probably caused by manipulation of the head during assisted ventilation.

Electrode Contact Artifact

Occasionally, an EEG electrode may come loose during the recording, or an electrode pad may be defective. In such cases, the resulting activity may be totally artifactual. An example is shown in the top (L) portion of Figure 8–9C, where artifactual activity on the left side persists past the end of the EEG seizure recorded from the intact leads on the right side of the head, as indicated by the arrow in the lower (R) portion of the figure. This example also demonstrates why the redundancy offered by two-channel recording offers an advantage over using a single EEG channel.

Electrocardiographic Artifact

An additional common type of artifact, particularly with a mastoid reference electrode, relates to the electrocardiogram. The practitioner should take care to avoid mistaking the usually rhythmic ECG or pulse artifact for continued seizure activity. However, this is generally not a difficult distinction because the ECG signal is typically low in amplitude, and its identity can be verified by checking the temporal relationship with the patient's pulse or ECG monitor signal. The ECG artifact is generally not apparent until the period of postictal flattening, when EEG activity is relatively suppressed. An example of postictal ECG artifact is shown in Figure 8–9D. One can see clear evidence of deflections in the EEG channel that are time-locked to the QRS complex in the ECG channel.

Ictal EEG Interpretation

The physician should be able to assess the EEG recording to determine whether a seizure has occurred and, if so, when it has ended. Several strategies for making these determinations are discussed in the following sections.

Determination of Seizure End Point

The seizure end point is defined as the point at which the last drop in amplitude occurs in the EEG signal following the onset of the seizure. Unfortunately, in practice, one cannot use this definition to determine the seizure end point unequivocally. For one to identify the final drop in amplitude, the patient would need to be monitored forever. Another challenge is that sometimes the seizure ends so gradually that one cannot discern a discrete end point (Krystal and Weiner 1995). However, by implementing a series of strategies, the clinician generally can identify the seizure end point without significant difficulty.

- *"When in doubt, play it out."* Because of the possibility that further evolution of the EEG activity may occur, the clinician should continue to record data if at all uncertain that the seizure has ended (see Figure 8–10).
- *Observe at least 10 seconds of data beyond the apparent end of the seizure.* This practice will lower the chances of selecting as the end point a decrease in amplitude that is not the final one. It will also greatly decrease the likelihood that seizure activity will resume after what is believed to be the end of the seizure. Resumption of seizure activity has been observed after periods as long as 5 seconds of what appears to be definitive postictal activity (see Figure 8–8, earlier in chapter).
- *Remember that the seizure is very likely to have ended if a period of > 5 seconds of EEG data is observed in at least one channel where the amplitude remains < 80 µV.* This rough rule of thumb is a corollary to the observation that the longest period of apparent postictal activity after which resumption of seizure activity has occurred is approximately 5 seconds. The 80-µV amplitude threshold should be considered approximate; the clinician should watch for a high degree of postictal suppression of EEG activity that creates the appearance of a flat or nearly flat electroencephalogram when the gain has been set as recommended in the section "Setting the Display and Printout Gain," earlier in this chapter. This strategy is useful for differentiating postictal EEG activity, during which there are intermittent slow-waves (a relatively common pattern), from ongoing ictal EEG activity. This strategy is also useful for identifying the end point when the electroencephalogram shows a great degree of artifact, which is often intermittently present postictally, such as occurs due to efforts to ventilate the patient.

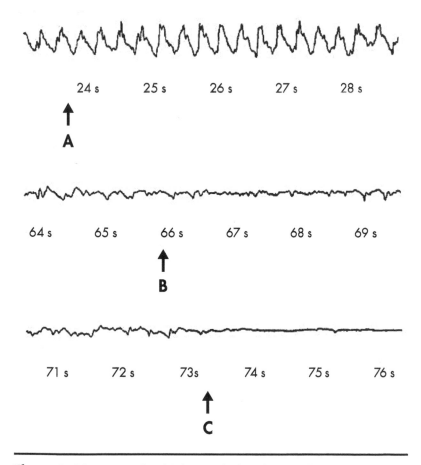

Figure 8–10.   Example of "when in doubt, play it out" strategy.

s = second.
(A) Ongoing seizure activity. (B) Significant drop in amplitude that was *not* the end of the seizure. (C) Actual seizure end point.

- *Watch for the immediate prestimulus EEG pattern to return; the point at which this occurs is the end point of the seizure.*
- *After identifying that the seizure has ended, work backward from the end of the data toward the beginning to determine the end point.* The clinician should

record data until certain that the seizure is over and then identify the end point as the first nonartifactual transition in the signal encountered when reading the data from the end back toward the beginning of the recording. This strategy is a standardized means of determining the end point when a very gradual transition occurs from the ictal to postictal pattern, as shown earlier in Figure 8–7.

- *If the patient initiates spontaneous movement or efforts to breathe, consider the seizure to be over.*
- *If artifact may be hindering the capacity to determine the seizure end point, consider asking that ventilation and other patient manipulations be suspended for 5–10 seconds.* This strategy will either allow the seizure end point to be determined or establish that such factors are not affecting signal quality.

Figures 8–5 and 8–6A illustrate cases in which well-defined ictal activity undergoes an abrupt transition into a relatively flat postictal baseline. In contrast, in Figure 8–6B, a similarly apparent abrupt end point is followed by a pattern of irregular slowing without flattening; this is an example of a situation in which the practitioner should continue to monitor the electroencephalogram to see whether this activity disappears into a much flatter baseline. Figures 8–7 and 8–10 provide examples in which playing out more data established that a significant drop in amplitude was not the seizure end point but part of the transition period and followed by a subsequent further decrease in signal amplitude.

Determination of Seizure Activity

As discussed in "Ictal EEG Phases" earlier in this chapter, the EEG activity observed when a seizure has been elicited tends to consist of a series of stages, each of which comprises waveforms of characteristic appearance. In practice, however, these features are not useful for determining whether a seizure has occurred. One reason is that significant variability occurs in the degree to which these stages and the associated waveforms are manifest during seizures. Another confound is that the appearance of the immediate prestimulus electroencephalogram may at times be indistinguishable from that of the characteristic ictal waveforms (see Figure 8–11). The determination of whether a seizure has been elicited is best made by looking for either of two types of pat-

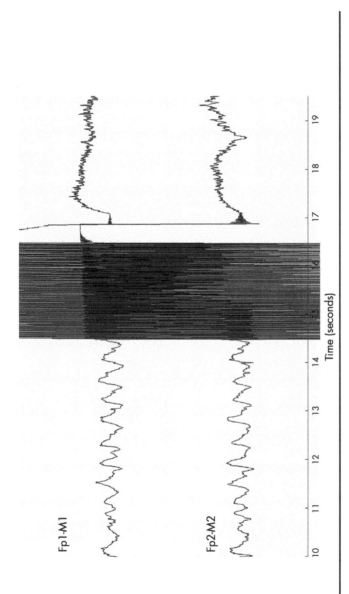

Figure 8–11. Electroencephalogram (EEG) data recorded just prior to and after the ECT stimulus (the dark band between 14 and 17 seconds).

Note that the prestimulus EEG resembles the pattern frequently seen in the clonic phase of seizures. In this case, the prestimulus pattern was caused by the effects of general anesthesia.

terns that are unique to seizure activity in this setting: 1) evolution in the dominant frequency in the electroencephalogram or 2) the addition of spikes to the prestimulus electroencephalogram, which then go away.

Evolution of the Dominant Frequency

Evolution from higher- to lower-frequency EEG activity is observed in all ECT seizures except those elicited with stimulus charge that is close to the patient's seizure threshold. Seizures of this type are illustrated in Figures 8–12 and 8–15A. Although the EEG signal generally comprises waveforms of multiple frequencies, the *dominant frequency* refers to the largest component present in the EEG signal. Looking for the dominant frequency is more useful than looking for characteristic waveforms when trying to distinguish EEG seizure activity from the EEG activity induced by anesthesia where no seizure has been elicited. This is because, although periods may occur during which the frequency content in the anesthesia electroencephalogram evolves, generally a sustained slowing of dominant frequency does not occur.

In some cases, all or nearly all of the evolution may take place in the first 5–10 seconds of the seizure, with sustained lower-frequency activity thereafter (see Figure 8–13). This pattern is helpful because it allows a rapid determination of whether there is a seizure; however, this is also the period of the seizure during which artifacts due to manipulations of the patient (e.g., removal of the mouth guard, initiation of ventilation) are most likely. As a result, optimal identification of seizure activity requires developing the skill of identifying the slowing in the dominant frequency component of the electroencephalogram despite the presence of artifacts.

In Figure 8–14, very-low-amplitude but high-frequency activity can be observed riding on top of the large waveforms generated by movement artifact and gradually evolve into higher-amplitude, lower-frequency activity, indicating the presence of a seizure in this patient. A "side-by-side" comparison of the segment of the EEG strip recorded in the first 10–20 seconds and of data from later in the recording may help in determining whether slowing in the dominant frequency has occurred.

Addition of Spikes, Which Then Go Away

When the stimulus intensity is barely suprathreshold, slowing of the dominant frequency in the electroencephalogram may not occur, may be extremely

A

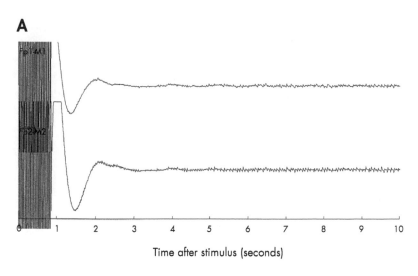

Time after stimulus (seconds)

B

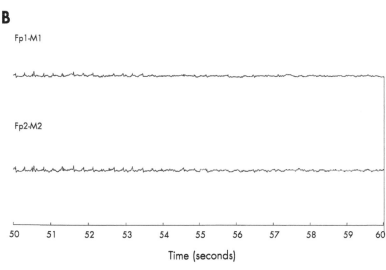

Time (seconds)

Figure 8–12.   Electroencephalogram recorded during threshold seizure.

(A) The beginning of the seizure is marked by relatively low-amplitude spike activity.
(B) The spike activity ceases with the transition to the termination phase of the seizure.

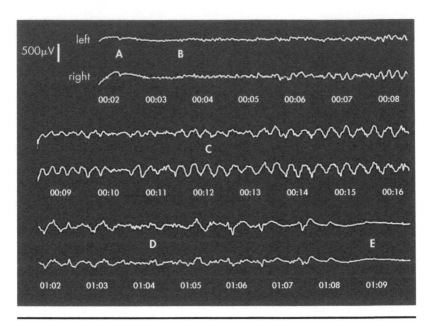

Figure 8–13.   Typical seizure with right unilateral ECT (d'Elia position).

This electroencephalogram illustrates early evolution of the seizure with a long slow-wave course. (A) Preictal activity. (B) Polyspike activity. (C) Polyspike and slow-wave activity. (D) Termination phase. (E) Postictal phase.

subtle, or may be delayed. The hallmark of seizures of this type is the addition of spikes to the EEG activity that was present immediately prior to the stimulus; these spikes then go away either in the transition to the termination phase or at the seizure end point. In this case, the most useful "side-by-side" comparison is between the EEG data recorded immediately prior to the stimulus and the data in the first 10–20 seconds after the stimulus. This spike pattern is easy to identify when the immediate prestimulus electroencephalogram is relatively low in amplitude. However, when higher-amplitude activity is present immediately prior to the stimulus, the addition of spikes may be more difficult to see, and a "side-by-side" comparison becomes a necessity. For seizures of this type, skill in detecting the seizure from reading the electroencephalogram is particularly important because the motor response is most likely to be absent.

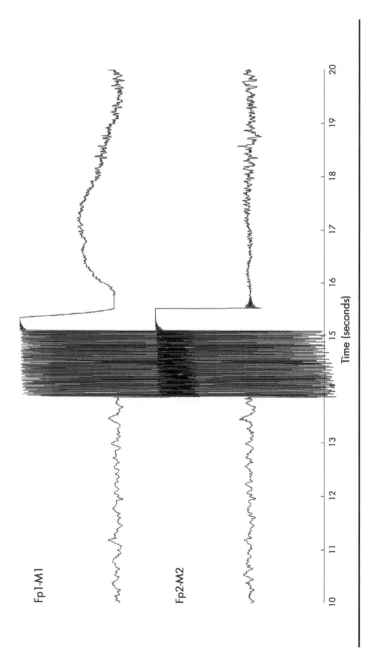

Figure 8–14. Low-amplitude but high-frequency seizure activity on top of large waveforms (motion artifact). The dark band from 14 to 15 seconds indicates the electrical stimulus.

Determination of Seizure Adequacy

Traditionally, achievement of an adequate seizure duration—for example, a 20-second motor response and/or a 25-second EEG response—has been assumed to be both necessary and sufficient to ensure therapeutic adequacy of ECT treatment (Ottosson 1960). However, multiple studies have established that right unilateral seizures that are marginally suprathreshold have poor therapeutic potency despite being of sufficient duration (Sackeim et al. 1987, 1993). This finding has led investigators to look for other measures of seizure adequacy, particularly those relating to the amplitude and shape of the ictal electroencephalogram (Krystal and Weiner 1994; Weiner et al. 1991).

For example, the low amplitude and poorly defined regularity of a barely suprathreshold seizure is depicted in Figure 8–12, which illustrates the ictal EEG response to a marginally intense ECT stimulus. In Figure 8–15A, a portion of a 35-second EEG seizure is shown. Because the patient's ictal EEG response was of much poorer quality than those responses obtained in previous treatments, and because no motor response was evident, the patient was restimulated at a higher intensity after a brief delay (see Chapter 11, "Managing the ECT Seizure"). The onset of seizure activity appears in Figure 8–15B, which shows the maximum EEG amplitude of the resulting 76-second seizure. (The motor convulsive response in this case was 54 seconds.) Viewing the differences between the two seizures, one can easily appreciate that both the amplitude and the regularity of the ictal EEG activity are substantially augmented by the more intensely (and possibly more therapeutic) suprathreshold stimulus.

Because such EEG differences can be categorized by quantitative features such as amplitude and frequency, the development of quantitative ictal EEG measures to predict the adequacy, or therapeutic potency, of ECT seizures has become of great contemporary interest (Krystal and Weiner 1994; Weiner et al. 1991). As noted in Chapter 5, "Clinical Applications," given that seizure threshold rises over the ECT course in an unpredictable fashion, such measures could also be used to predict how close to seizure threshold a stimulus was, thereby serving as an aid to future stimulus dosing (Krystal and Weiner 1995; Krystal et al. 1993). For example, barely suprathreshold (and presumably less effective) seizures tend to be lower in ictal amplitude, higher in postictal amplitude (less postictal suppression), and slower to develop patterns of ictal slowing (Krystal and Weiner 1995).

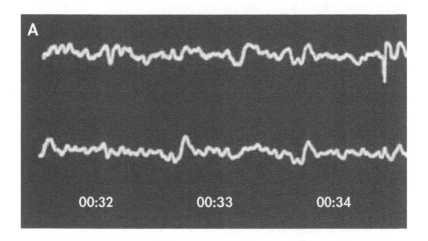

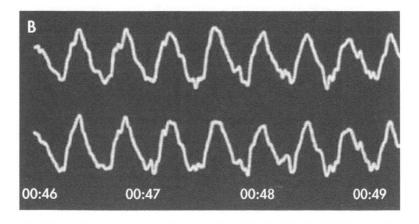

Figure 8–15.   Two seizures of markedly different amplitude and frequency in the same patient.

(A) Barely suprathreshold seizure showing poorly defined ictal activity. (B) A second seizure in the same patient, who was restimulated after a brief delay.

References

Krystal AD, Weiner RD: ECT seizure therapeutic adequacy. Convuls Ther 10:153–164, 1994

Krystal AD, Weiner RD: ECT seizure duration: reliability of manual and computer-automated determinations. Convuls Ther 11:158–169, 1995

Krystal AD, Weiner RD, McCall WV, et al: The effects of ECT stimulus dose and electrode placement on the ictal electroencephalogram: an intraindividual cross-over study. Biol Psychiatry 34:759–767, 1993

Liston EH, Guze BH, Baxter LR Jr, et al: Motor versus EEG seizure during ECT. Biol Psychiatry 24:94–96, 1988

Ottosson JO: Experimental studies of the mode of action of electroconvulsive therapy. Acta Psychiatr Scand 35(suppl):1–141, 1960

Sackeim HA, Decina P, Kanzler M, et al: Effects of electrode placement on the efficacy of titrated, low-dose ECT. Am J Psychiatry 144:1449–1455, 1987

Sackeim HA, Prudic J, Devanand DP, et al: Effects of stimulus intensity and electrode placement on the efficacy and cognitive effects of electroconvulsive therapy. N Engl J Med 328:839–846, 1993

Swartz CM, Abrams R: An auditory representation of ECT-induced seizures. Convuls Ther 2:125–128, 1986

Weiner RD, Coffey CE, Krystal AD: The monitoring and management of electrically induced seizures. Psychiatr Clin North Am 14:845–869, 1991

9

Cardiovascular Response

Andrew D. Krystal, M.D., M.S.

In addition to the cerebral electrophysiological changes produced by ECT, transient cardiovascular alterations also take place. This chapter focuses on the equipment generally used to monitor these changes and the physiological principles involved in these cardiovascular responses to ECT.

Monitoring Equipment

In ECT treatment and recovery settings, a variety of equipment is used to monitor the cardiovascular response of the patient before, during, and after the induced seizure (American Psychiatric Association 2001; Gaines and Rees 1992). Cardiac monitors used in such settings typically measure the patient's blood pressure, heart rate, and the heart's electrical activity; however, some older models may monitor only the heart's electrical activity and pulse, requiring the blood pressure to be taken manually. Many newer monitors can be programmed to check the blood pressure regularly or to sound an alert au-

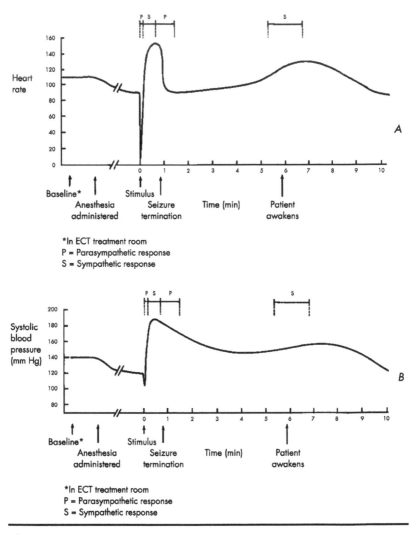

Figure 9–1.   ECT effects on heart rate (A) and systolic blood pressure (B).

tomatically if an abnormal beat or rhythm occurs. A pulse oximeter is used to assess continuously the oxygen saturation of the patient's blood. Oxygen levels between 95% and 100% indicate adequate oxygenation. This information is gathered with a lighted clip, generally attached to the patient's finger.

Acute Cardiovascular Response to ECT

Figure 9–1 schematically depicts the typical effects of ECT on heart rate and systolic blood pressure (Perrin 1961). Before anesthesia induction, both measures are often elevated because of the patient's anxiety. As the anesthetic agent takes effect, heart rate and blood pressure generally decrease, although the muscle relaxant succinylcholine may at least partially reverse this effect.

The ECT stimulus and the induced seizure both exert cardiovascular effects, primarily through the direct neuronal transmission from the hypothalamus to the heart via parasympathetic tracts (the vagus nerve) and sympathetic tracts (primarily in the spinal cord). The activation of the parasympathetic system causes a decrease in blood pressure and heart rate. The activation of the sympathetic system produces opposite effects: blood pressure, venous pressure, and heart rate increase, resulting in an overall acceleration of cardiac output.

The cardiovascular response pattern can best be described as a four-stage process, involving shifts from parasympathetic to sympathetic to parasympathetic to sympathetic phases (see Figure 9–1). Just after the electrical stimulus, the initial parasympathetic activation occurs, as a result of the direct stimulation of certain brain stem nuclei. This activation results in a drop in blood pressure and a transient sinus bradycardia or sinus asystole, which often lasts several seconds. Occasionally, sinus pauses have been observed to last 10 seconds or more. Figure 9–2A shows a sinus asystole of 6 seconds. At the patient's next treatment (Figure 9–2B), asystole was avoided by increasing the dose of the anticholinergic agent.

The initial parasympathetic response is immediately followed by a sympathetic discharge, in which blood pressure and heart rate rise dramatically. This sympathetic surge is usually absent in the case of a missed seizure, leaving the parasympathetic effects unopposed. The ictal tachycardia continues until the end of the clonic phase, when the parasympathetic system is reactivated. The reactivation is often accompanied by an abrupt drop in the cardiac rate, which may sometimes present as bradycardia, as seen in Figure 9–3. These events are then followed by a second phase of sympathetic hyperactivity upon awakening. Both the final parasympathetic and final sympathetic phases are usually less prominent than their initial counterparts, although the presence of a postictal agitation potentiates the last sympathetic discharge. Eventually,

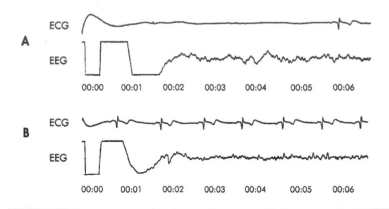

Figure 9–2.   Sinus asystole and response to anticholinergic pretreatment.

A shows a sinus asystole of 6 seconds. At the patient's next treatment (B), asystole was avoided by increasing the dose of the anticholinergic agent.

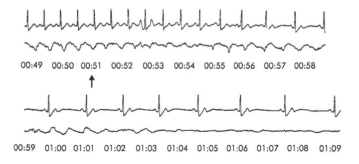

Figure 9–3.   Bradycardia during parasympathetic reactivation.

The upper portion shows ictal tachycardia (about 120/second) followed by postictal bradycardia (about 38/second). The arrow denotes the end of motor convulsion.

as the patient becomes fully alert, blood pressure and heart rate should return to their baseline levels. The effects of a sympatholytic agent or other drug with similar properties given at the time of ECT may persist, however.

During the seizure, the electrocardiogram may demonstrate peaked T waves (Khoury and Benedetti 1989). This is a benign phenomenon due to the electrical

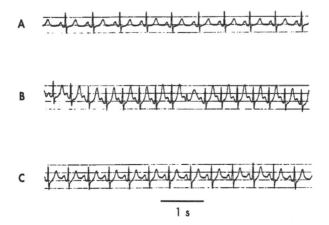

Figure 9–4. Peaked T waves.

(A) Prestimulus (baseline); (B) early ictal; (C) early postictal.

stimulation of brain stem centers important to cardiac polarization. T wave amplitude typically normalizes soon after completion of the seizure (see Figure 9–4).

In patients with functioning indwelling pacemakers and defibrillators, ECT is quite safe electrically (Alexopoulos 1980; Pinski and Trohman 1995), with the exception of transcutaneous devices or internal wiring that has been disrupted. (In the latter case, the pacemaker would be inoperative.) For that matter, the protective effects of these devices on cardiac rhythm are such that the patient is actually safer receiving ECT with them than without them. Still, the autonomic changes that take place during a seizure may result in a phasic activation and/or deactivation of some older demand pacemakers (see Figure 9–5). For this reason, it is generally prudent to convert such devices temporarily to a fixed mode before each anesthesia induction; this can be done by placing a magnet on the skin overlying the pacemaker. However, this procedure may not be necessary with more modern pacemakers (this should be determined by a cardiology consultation; see Chapter 3, "Patient Referral and Evaluation"). A similar procedure is used in patients with some implanted defibrillators to ensure that these autonomic surges do not inadvertently trigger activation of the device; again, however, some of the more recent devices may not require this action.

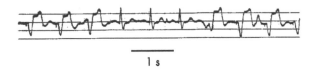

1 s

Figure 9–5. Intermittent activation of demand pacemaker.

Signal artifacts, which were noted in Chapter 8 to be a problem with ictal electroencephalographic recordings, may also present difficulties with electrocardiogram interpretation, as seen in Figure 9–6. Figure 9–6A shows a case in which movement artifact renders the determination of cardiac rhythm difficult. A more extreme example is depicted in Figure 9–6B, where there is probably poor electrocardiographic (ECG) electrode contact with the skin. Rarely, the ECG signal may be completely blocked, as can be seen in Figure 9–6C. For obvious reasons, it is important to discriminate readily between this type of artifact and a true cardiac arrest; this can be done by feeling for the pulse or by auscultating the heart.

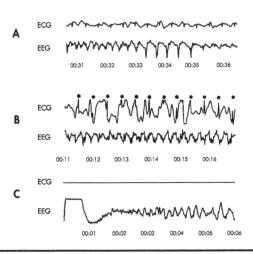

Figure 9–6. Electrocardiographic (ECG) artifact. recorded with ECT.

(A) Baseline sway; (B) Gross movement artifact (dots indicate locations of QRS complex); (C) total loss of ECG signal.

References

Alexopoulos GS: ECT and cardiac patients with pacemakers. Am J Psychiatry 137:1111–1112, 1980

American Psychiatric Association: The Practice of Electroconvulsive Therapy: Recommendations for Treatment, Training, and Privileging (A Task Force Report of the American Psychiatric Association), 2nd Edition. Washington, DC, American Psychiatric Publishing, 2001

Gaines GY, Rees DI: Anesthetic considerations for electroconvulsive therapy. South Med J 85:469–482, 1992

Khoury GF, Benedetti C: T-wave changes associated with electroconvulsive therapy. Anesth Analg 69:677–679, 1989

Perrin GM: Cardiovascular aspects of electric shock therapy. Acta Psychiatr Neurol Scand 36:7–44, 1961

Pinski SL, Trohman RG: Implantable cardioverter-defibrillators: implications for the nonelectrophysiologist. Ann Intern Med 122:770–777, 1995

PART 4

Treatment Course

10

Adverse Effects

Mehul V. Mankad, M.D.
Richard D. Weiner, M.D., Ph.D.

As with any acute medical intervention, ECT procedures carry some risk. These risks are associated with the induction of general anesthesia, the seizure and convulsion, the interaction between concomitant medications and ECT, and other aspects of the ECT procedure. The most common side effects involve cognitive changes, transient cardiovascular alterations, and general somatic complaints. Proper diagnosis, pre-ECT evaluation, and the use of modified ECT techniques have significantly decreased the incidence and severity of adverse effects. As part of the decision to refer a patient for ECT, the clinician must consider each case on its own merits, weighing both risks and benefits. Such risk-benefit considerations are discussed further in Chapter 11, "Managing the ECT Seizure"; Chapter 12, "Index ECT"; and Chapter 13, "Maintenance ECT."

Table 10–1.   Medical conditions associated with increased risk from ECT

Space-occupying intracerebral lesion (tumor, hematoma, etc.)
Other condition causing increased intracranial pressure
Recent myocardial infarction
Recent intracerebral hemorrhage
Unstable vascular aneurysm or malformation
Pheochromocytoma
High anesthesia risk (American Society of Anesthesiologists [ASA] class 4 or 5)

Source.   American Psychiatric Association 2001.

Contraindications

According to the American Psychiatric Association (2001), ECT has no absolute contraindications. However, some conditions pose a relatively high risk. As summarized in Table 10–1, these include space-occupying intracerebral lesions (except small, slow-growing tumors without edema or other mass effect), other conditions causing increased intracranial pressure, recent myocardial infarction with substantially compromised cardiac function, recent intracerebral hemorrhage, unstable vascular aneurysms or malformations, and pheochromocytoma (American Psychiatric Association 2001). If treatment with ECT becomes necessary on a lifesaving basis for a patient with one of these conditions, antecedent risks can generally be minimized to some extent pharmacologically (Weiner and Coffey 1993).

Mortality Rate

Despite what can be perceived as the invasive nature of ECT, the overall mortality rate from ECT in a general population of patients is extremely low, estimated at 2–10 per 100,000 patients (0.0001%) (Shiwach et al. 2001). This is roughly the same ratio as for the induction of brief general anesthesia itself. Nuttall et al. (2004) found no ECT-related deaths in a 13-year sample of 17,394 treatments. Some data suggest that patients who receive ECT have a lower mortality rate due to nonpsychiatric causes of death than do patients with psychiatric illness who do not receive ECT (Munk-Olsen et al. 2007).

However, significant risk factors (e.g., severe coronary artery disease, unstable vascular anomalies, greatly compromised respiratory function, overall high anesthetic risk) clearly increase the risk of death with ECT. This relationship should be kept in mind, not only in regard to estimation of risk levels, but also in terms of informed consent (see Chapter 3, "Patient Referral and Evaluation").

Cognitive Changes

Cognitive changes are often the most notable and most distressing side effects of ECT. The clinician should keep in mind a couple of facts about cognitive changes: First, depressive episodes themselves are often accompanied by profound cognitive changes, which are sometimes severe enough to present as dementia (pseudodementia). In such cases, a successful response to ECT may actually be associated with at least a subjective improvement in cognitive status. Second, cognitive change is not equivalent to structural brain damage. Extensive research has found no relationship between ECT and brain damage (Agelink et al. 2001; Scalia et al. 2007; Zachrisson et al. 2000). Some animal models and in vitro studies indicate that ECT may actually increase neuronal sprouting and synaptic strength rather than lead to cellular toxicity (Duman and Vaidya 1998). Interestingly, these changes are in the opposite direction to those reported to occur in the context of animal models of depressive illness.

Three types of cognitive impairment, discussed below, may be observed with ECT: postictal disorientation, interictal confusion, and amnesia (anterograde and retrograde memory disturbances).

Postictal Disorientation

Because ECT induces seizure activity, all patients experience some transient postictal disorientation, lasting from a few minutes to a few hours, following awakening from the ECT treatment. Having received general anesthesia likely contributes to this disorientation. A variety of factors can affect the severity of ECT-related cognitive dysfunction (see Table 10–2), including the postictal confusional state.

Most patients do not experience the postictal cognitive changes following a seizure as a significant disturbance and, in fact, are often amnestic for the im-

Table 10–2. Factors that may increase cognitive side effects

Factor	Effect
Stimulus waveform	Sine wave>brief pulse
Stimulus intensity	High>low
Electrode placement	Bilateral>unilateral
Number of treatments	Many>few
Frequency of treatments	Frequent>infrequent
Patient age	Older>younger
Preexisting cognitive deficiencies	Present>absent

mediate postictal time period. Typically, treatment involves providing reassurance and support and helping the patient avoid cognitive demands during the acute postictal period, although postictal sedation with a short-acting benzodiazepine (e.g., midazolam) or intravenous haloperidol may sometimes be necessary if the patient becomes agitated.

Interictal Confusion

Occasionally, postictal confusion may not fully disappear and, when severe, may develop into an interictal confusional state or delirium. This phenomenon, which is uncommon, is affected by the same factors as postictal disorientation (see Table 10–2). When present, interictal confusion is cumulative over the ECT course, but it rapidly disappears over a period of days following the conclusion of treatments.

The sudden onset of an interictal confusional state, particularly within hours or even days after the most recent ECT treatment, is a cause for concern and must be quickly assessed. A variety of factors may be involved, including recent medication changes (e.g., withdrawal effects), substance abuse or withdrawal, acute exposure to toxic substances (accidental or purposeful), nonconvulsive status epilepticus, or acute dissociative state. If nonconvulsive status is considered an emergency, an electroencephalogram should be ordered.

Memory Impairment

Amnesia often occurs with ECT and varies considerably in both severity and persistence, particularly with respect to the patient's self-perception of memory function (Dukakis and Tye 2006; Vamos 2008). Memory disturbances consist of both retrograde amnesia (difficulty in recalling information learned before the ECT course) and anterograde amnesia (difficulty in retaining newly learned information) (Fraser et al 2008; Ingram et al. 2008). The same factors that affect the extent of postictal confusion (see Table 10–2) also affect the likelihood, severity, and persistence of memory deficits. Indeed, the duration of postictal disorientation is highly correlated with the extent and persistence of retrograde amnesia following ECT. Retrograde amnesia is most severe for events occurring closer in time to the ECT. Less commonly, material from more remote periods may be affected, particularly when large numbers of bilateral ECT treatments have been administered.

Objective memory testing measures indicate that anterograde amnesia typically disappears over a period of days to weeks after completion of the ECT course. Other such studies report that retrograde amnesia also significantly improves, but sometimes over a longer time period. Retrograde amnesia may not completely resolve, however, especially recall of the time period covering the ECT course and, to a lesser degree, the weeks and months before the ECT. Furthermore, retrograde amnesia with ECT has been described as "spotty" in temporal distribution and similar to that observed with other types of biologically mediated retrograde amnesia. In some cases, the memory traces are not truly "lost," but rather are more difficult to access from storage.

Irrespective of studies based on objective testing results, some individuals who have received ECT report that their ability to remember old, or even new, material never returns to "normal" following ECT (Dukakis and Tye 2006; Feliu et al. 2008; Vamos 2008). The etiology of this phenomenon is unclear, and objective memory testing does not generally provide corroboration. This subjective sense of decreased memory capability has been postulated to be due to any of several factors:

- A sensitization to normal forgetting following the transient organic amnesia that often accompanies the ECT treatment course
- Residual and/or recurrent symptoms related to the condition for which ECT was used
- Concurrent medication use or substance abuse
- Comorbid brain disease
- A conversion type of syndrome

- Psychological reinforcement of transient organic losses (secondary gain)
- An idiosyncratic neurobiological effect

Interestingly, self-ratings of memory change shortly following ECT appear to be more highly correlated with therapeutic outcome than with the results of objective memory testing. This is not unexpected, given the fact that upon recovery from an acute depressive episode, almost everything seems better.

Differences of opinion exist regarding the utility of routine memory testing before, shortly after, and months after receiving an index ECT course (American Psychiatric Association 2001; Porter et al. 2008). Certainly, routine "bedside" assessment of cognitive function is part of the mental status exam done during the pre-ECT evaluation. Theoretically, it would be good to be able to have an objective measure of baseline memory function prior to ECT and also to be able to determine whether and to what degree amnesia is present following ECT and whether persistent memory problems are reported. Indeed, some ECT programs do use formal testing, at least for anterograde amnesia (for which numerous standardized instruments exist—primarily based on the patient's ability to retain newly learned information over a period of distraction). However, in practice, such testing of ECT patients is problematic for a variety of reasons:

- Cognitive testing of severely depressed patient is sometimes invalid.
- Testing may be time consuming and difficult to schedule for a patient being worked up for ECT.
- Third-party carriers may not be willing to pay for routine testing.

If routine testing is desired, including some sort of global self-rating instrument would be useful because patients' complaints of memory dysfunction following ECT are related more to self-perception than to scores on a test battery.

The physiological mechanisms underlying ECT-related amnesia are unclear, although recent imaging studies suggest that both mesial temporal and frontal structures may be involved (Nobler and Sackeim 2008). A large number of pharmacological agents have been investigated as means to diminish the cognitive deficits associated with electrically induced seizures, but so far none has proved successful on a consistent basis (Pigot et al. 2008). However, abundant evidence indicates that modification of technical factors related to the ECT can significantly diminish the severity and/or persistence of ECT-related amnesia (Prudic 2008). These efforts include the following:

- Switching from bitemporal to unilateral nondominant stimulus electrode placement
- Switching from brief pulse to ultra-brief pulse stimuli
- Decreasing stimulus intensity (as long as intensity remains sufficiently over seizure threshold)
- Decreasing the frequency of index ECT treatments to two or even one per week
- Ensuring that the number of ECT treatments in the index course is not greater than that required to produce a therapeutic plateau
- Discontinuing or decreasing dosage of any standing medications that may themselves have an adverse impact on memory function

Cardiovascular Complications

Cardiovascular complications are the main cause of mortality and serious morbidity with ECT, although most such complications are minor (Weiner and Coffey 1993; Zielinski et al. 1996). During the seizure and acute postictal period, both the sympathetic and parasympathetic autonomic systems are sequentially stimulated (see Chapter 9, "Cardiovascular Response"). Activation of the sympathetic system increases heart rate, blood pressure, and myocardial oxygen consumption, placing an increased demand on the cardiovascular system. Indeed, ECT itself has been shown to induce peak heart rates in the range of 160–180 beats per minute, effectively replicating a pharmacologically induced cardiac stress test (Swartz and Shen 2007). Activation of the parasympathetic system causes a transient reduction in cardiac rate.

These changes in heart rate and cardiac output challenge the cardiovascular system, occasionally giving rise to transient arrhythmias and, in susceptible individuals, transient ischemic changes. During the sympathetically mediated tachycardia, ventricular arrhythmias may arise, particularly in those patients with preexisting cardiac ischemia. Substantial transient hypertension also occurs during the sympathetic discharge (frequently with systolic increase of 50 mm Hg or more) and may further raise the risk of ischemia in patients who have preexisting hypertension or whose ability to maintain a markedly increased cardiac output is diminished. Interestingly, however, the risk of a hypertensive intracerebral bleed during ECT is quite low. The risk of embolic stroke after ECT is also extremely rare (Lee 2006). During parasympathetic stimulation, cardiac arrhythmias, such as bradycardia, premature ventricular contractions, or sinus arrest, may be seen. In most patients, these arrhythmias are transient and occur without substantial sequelae.

The risks of cardiac arrhythmias, ischemia, and hypertension are greatly diminished by the use of oxygenation before and during the seizure, and these risks can be lowered further in susceptible patients by pretreatment with appropriate medications (see Chapter 6, "Anesthetics and Other Medications"). For example, administration of anticholinergic medications before the ECT treatment will lower the occurrence and severity of parasympathetically induced arrhythmias. Similarly, pretreatment with beta-blockers or a variety of other agents can diminish sympathetically mediated arrhythmias and hypertension, whereas antianginal medications exert a protective effect in those at risk for ischemic changes.

Other factors that have potential cardiotoxic effects during ECT include anoxia (which can be prevented by adequate ventilation and muscular relaxation), the rapid increase in serum potassium induced by the action of succinylcholine (highest in patients with widespread muscular rigidity or damage), and rare idiosyncratic reactions to generalized anesthesia.

Other Adverse Effects

General somatic complaints (e.g., headaches, nausea, muscle soreness) are usually minor but are frequent side effects of ECT. Headaches, generalized muscle soreness, and jaw pain are the most common side effects, usually lasting up to several hours, but occasionally longer. Headaches with ECT are believed to be usually related to the superficial vasodilation associated with the direct electrical effects of the stimulus and are most common with the initial treatment in a series. In patients who routinely have post-ECT headaches, analgesics may be given prophylactically before (if oral) or at the time of (if intravenous) ECT. Generalized muscle pain is usually caused by fasciculations associated with the depolarizing action of the muscle relaxant succinylcholine that is routinely used with ECT. Again, prophylaxis with analgesics is the most common management tool.

During the electrical stimulus in ECT, clenching of the jaw may occur as a result of direct stimulation of the masseter muscles. Because of the muscular contractions, dental appliances (e.g., dentures) should be removed before treatment (McCall et al. 1992). A soft bite block or other such device is used to prevent injury to the tongue or teeth, but dental problems or damage to soft oral tissues may occur in patients with loose or jagged teeth. Modification of this procedure or removal of such teeth will help prevent such problems.

A small percentage of depressed patients with bipolar disorder can switch into a manic or mixed state when treated with ECT, just as can occur with antidepressant medications. This switch may be managed by either continuing the ECT course or stopping ECT and administering an antimanic agent. The action taken usually depends on whether overt mania is present, in which case it is preferable (though also counterintuitive to some degree) to continue the ECT.

References

Agelink MW, Andrich J, Postert T, et al: Relation between electroconvulsive therapy, cognitive side effects, neuron specific enolase, and protein S-100. J Neurol Neurosurg Psychiatry 71:394–396, 2001

American Psychiatric Association: The Practice of Electroconvulsive Therapy: Recommendations for Treatment, Training, and Privileging (A Task Force Report of the American Psychiatric Association), 2nd Edition. Washington, DC, American Psychiatric Publishing, 2001

Dukakis K, Tye L: Shock: The Healing Power of Electroconvulsive Therapy. New York, Avery, 2006

Duman RS, Vaidya VA: Molecular and cellular actions of chronic electroconvulsive seizures. J ECT 14:181–193, 1998

Feliu M, Edwards CL, Sudhakar S, et al: Neuropsychological effects and attitudes in patients following electroconvulsive therapy. Neuropsychiatr Dis Treat 4:613–617, 2008

Fraser LM, O'Carroll RE, Ebmeier KP: The effect of electroconvulsive therapy on autobiographical memory: a systematic review. J ECT 24:10–17, 2008

Ingram A, Saling MM, Schweitzer I: Cognitive side effects of brief pulse electroconvulsive therapy: a review. J ECT 24:3–9, 2008

Lee K: Acute embolic stroke after electroconvulsive therapy. J ECT 22:67–69, 2006

McCall WV, Minneman SA, Weiner RD, et al: Dental pathology in ECT patients prior to treatment. Convuls Ther 8:19–24, 1992

Munk-Olsen T, Laursen TM, Videbech P, et al: All-cause mortality among recipients of electroconvulsive therapy. Br J Psychiatry 190:435–439, 2007

Nobler MS, Sackeim HA: Neurobiological correlates of the cognitive side effects of electroconvulsive therapy. J ECT 24:40–45, 2008

Nuttall GA, Bowersox MR, Douglass SB, et al: Morbidity and mortality in the use of electroconvulsive therapy. J ECT 20:237–241, 2004

Pigot M, Andrade C, Loo C: Pharmacological attenuation of electroconvulsive therapy–induced cognitive deficits: theoretical background and clinical findings. J ECT 24:57–67, 2008

Porter RJ, Douglas K, Knight RG: Monitoring of cognitive effects during a course of electroconvulsive therapy: recommendations for clinical practice. J ECT 24:25–34, 2008

Prudic J: Strategies to minimize cognitive side effects with ECT: aspects of ECT technique. J ECT 24:46–51, 2008

Scalia J, Lisanby SH, Dwork AJ, et al: Neuropathologic examination after 91 ECT treatments in a 92-year-old woman with late-onset depression. J ECT 23:96–98, 2007

Shiwach RS, Reid WH, Carmody TJ: An analysis of reported deaths following electroconvulsive therapy in Texas, 1993–1998. Psychiatr Serv 52:1095–1097, 2001

Swartz CM, Shen WW: ECT generalized seizure drives heart rate above treadmill stress test maximum. J ECT 23:71–74, 2007

Vamos M: The cognitive side effects of modern ECT: Patient experience or objective measurement. J ECT 24:18–23, 2008

Weiner RD, Coffey CE: Electroconvulsive therapy in the medical and neurologic patient, in Psychiatric Care of the Medical Patient. Edited by Stoudemire A, Fogel BS. New York, Oxford University Press, 1993, pp 207–224

Zachrisson OC, Balldin J, Ekman R, et al: No evident neuronal damage after electroconvulsive therapy. Psychiatry Res 96:157–165, 2000

Zielinski RJ, Roose SP, Devanand DP, et al: Cardiovascular complications of ECT in depressed patients with cardiac disease. Am J Psychiatry 150:904–909, 1996

11

Managing the ECT Seizure

Andrew D. Krystal, M.D., M.S.

Ensuring an adequate seizure is an essential component of the ECT procedure. The practitioner's response to missed and other inadequate seizures must be both rapid and effective to ensure that an adequate seizure is eventually obtained. Various seizure augmentation strategies are often useful in this regard. Similarly, the practitioner must be aware of the need to manage prolonged seizures, which can be associated with adverse sequelae. These are the topics covered in this chapter.

Missed Seizures

Missed seizures are detected when no motor and ictal evidence of seizure activity is seen following the electrical stimulus (Weiner et al. 1991). Although some muscular contraction usually occurs during the period of electrical stimulation, this should not be mistaken for seizure activity, nor should the physician mistake movement artifacts or anesthesia-related activity on the electroencephalographic (EEG) tracing as evidence of seizure activity (see Figures 8–9B and 8–14 in Chapter 8, "Ictal Electroencephalographic Response"). Finally, because the onset of seizure activity may be delayed (particularly when the stimulus is close to seizure threshold), the practitioner should wait 10–15 seconds following the stimulus before concluding that a missed seizure has occurred.

Factors that can play a role in the occurrence of missed or inadequate seizures include insufficient stimulus intensity (including premature termination of the stimulus by releasing pressure from the stimulus button of the ECT device); poor stimulus electrode contact with the skin; a patient's high intrinsic seizure threshold; hypercarbia (i.e., increased carbon dioxide levels, usually due to hypoventilation); a rise in seizure threshold, which often occurs over the ECT treatment course (Krystal et al. 1998, 2000); and a patient's taking medications with anticonvulsant properties (including the barbiturate anesthetic used with ECT).

After a missed seizure has been diagnosed, the physician should first attempt to ascertain the etiology of the problem. If the cause of the missed seizure was the premature termination of the stimulus, the patient should be restimulated at the original stimulus dosage. If poor stimulus electrode contact with the skin was believed to be the cause (e.g., excessively high dynamic impedance), then better contact should be attempted and the patient restimulated at the same stimulus intensity. If a malfunction in the ECT device is suspected, no further stimulation should be carried out until the problem is corrected. For other causes, the patient should be restimulated at a higher stimulus dosage.

When a missed seizure occurs, the patient should be restimulated within 20–30 seconds, using a 25%–125% increase in stimulus intensity (American Psychiatric Association 2001). Given that patients receiving ECT generally have a relatively urgent need for a therapeutic response, the practitioner should ensure that an adequate seizure is eventually obtained, if at all possible.

If a restimulation is required, the physician must make certain that the patient remains adequately anesthetized, that the patient's muscles remain relaxed, and that the staff member in contact with the patient's head is ready. Signs that the patient is regaining consciousness include purposeful movements or a sudden increase in heart rate before the stimulation. Asking the patient to move his or her cuffed foot may help in determining if the patient is waking up. In such cases, the physician should immediately administer an additional modest dose of the anesthetic agent (e.g., methohexital 10–30 mg iv). Proper relaxation can be reassessed by examining the deep tendon reflexes or the withdrawal reflex. In this regard, the resumption of spontaneous breathing is a sign that relaxation is suboptimal, so an additional small dose of relaxant agent should be administered.

After successfully eliciting a seizure, the physician should review possible causes of the missed seizure. Particular attention should be paid to any relevant changes in the patient's pharmacological regimen and also to a reevaluation of the dosage of anesthetic agent. If the source of the missed seizure is not identified, the stimulus intensity for the next treatment should be at least what was successful in inducing a seizure in the treatment just completed. If the stimulus parameters are at the maximum amount allowed by the ECT device, strategies for decreasing seizure threshold should be considered (see "Seizure Augmentation" below).

Inadequate Seizures

The consensus regarding how to assess seizure adequacy is not as great as that concerning what represents a missed seizure (Weiner et al. 1991). As noted in Chapter 8, practitioners have traditionally used a motor or EEG seizure end point criterion, typically around 20–25 seconds. However, some data suggested not only that some short seizures may be therapeutically adequate, but that some seizures of "adequate" duration—for example, those associated with barely suprathreshold pulse unilateral treatments (Sackeim et al. 1987, 1993)— are not therapeutic. Therefore, since the 1990s, research in this area has focused on the use of alternative ictal EEG measures of treatment adequacy— for example, the degree of suppression of EEG activity occurring at the end of the seizure (postictal suppression) (Krystal and Weiner 1994, 1995). In addition to electrophysiological measures, certain characteristics of the neuroendocrine response to the seizure (most notably prolactin [Robin et al. 1985]) have been considered, although these have not yet provided clinically meaningful measures of predicting therapeutic adequacy.

In general, inadequate seizures appear to result from the same factors as missed seizures, and the same clinical procedures should be followed as with missed seizures, except that restimulation should be delayed for 30–60 seconds because of the presence of a transient refractory period. During this time, the physician should pay attention to ensuring that adequate anesthetic and relaxant effects are still present.

An algorithm for management of ECT-induced seizures, incorporating these recommendations, is provided in Figure 11–1.

Seizure Augmentation

Evidence suggests that missed or inadequate seizures occurring at maximum stimulus intensity decrease the likelihood that the patient will respond to treatment. When these phenomena occur, efforts should be directed at decreasing the seizure threshold, increasing the seizure duration, or both (Krystal et al. 2000). Presently, four methods of seizure enhancement are commonly used: decreasing the anesthetic dosage (if possible and if the agent used has anticonvulsant properties), hyperventilation (inducing hypocarbia), caffeine (and other adenosine receptor antagonists), and ketamine anesthesia (Weiner et al. 1991).

Hyperventilation

Substantially decreasing the patient's carbon dioxide level results in an approximately 100% increase in seizure duration (Bergsholm et al. 1984), although the seizure threshold itself may not be affected. Inducing hypocarbia is most easily achieved by hyperventilating the patient. The anesthesiologist should apply slow, deep respirations, beginning before the anesthesia induction and continuing until an adequate seizure duration has been obtained. At the same time, care should be taken to avoid continuation of the hyperventilation much past this point, because the resulting hypocarbic state will delay the resumption of spontaneous breathing.

Caffeine

Caffeine is another seizure augmentation strategy (Coffey et al. 1990; Weiner et al. 1991). It is available in the United States for parenteral use as 2-mL ampules containing 500 mg of caffeine sodium benzoate, which is equivalent to about 250 mg of caffeine. The usual initial dosage of caffeine is 250 mg infused intravenously, over a 20-second period, 2 minutes before the anes-

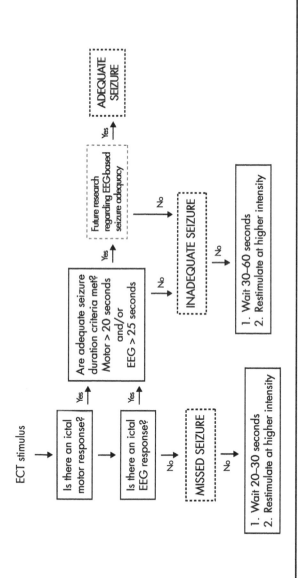

Figure 11–1. Algorithm for management of ECT seizure adequacy.

EEG=electroencephalogram.

thetic is administered. Caffeine typically increases seizure duration by 100%, although tolerance eventually develops. Seizure threshold itself does not appear to be affected (McCall et al. 1993). Dosages up to 1,000 mg (2,000 mg of caffeine sodium benzoate) may be used by giving increments of 125–250 mg per trial.

Because caffeine may cause a transient rise in blood pressure and pulse, either it should be avoided or lower dosages should be considered for patients with a history of cardiovascular problems. Caffeine may also cause an increase in anxiety and agitation, particularly in patients prone to such states. Interestingly, some data have suggested that caffeine may potentiate not only seizure duration but therapeutic response as well, and that caffeine may also diminish adverse cognitive effects associated with ECT (Calev et al. 1993).

Changes to Anesthetic Regimen

Because barbiturate anesthetics cause an increase in seizure threshold and a decrease in seizure duration, seizures may also be augmented by decreasing the dosage of barbiturate or other anticonvulsant anesthetics and substituting a different anesthetic agent, ketamine, for all or part of the dosage (Brewer et al. 1972). Because ketamine does not increase seizure threshold, switching to it is associated with a functional decrease in seizure threshold as well as an increase in seizure duration. For this reason, ketamine is specifically indicated in cases of missed seizures that cannot be managed by 1) increasing the stimulus intensity, 2) decreasing the dosage of the routine anesthetic agent, or 3) decreasing or stopping other medications with anticonvulsant properties. Because ketamine is occasionally associated with a transient emergence psychosis (relatively more likely if it is not possible to elicit a seizure), and because the drug has a higher cardiotoxic effect than barbiturate anesthetics, it is usually reserved for the management of high seizure thresholds rather than short seizure durations (Krystal et al. 2003). (For dosing instructions, see Chapter 6, "Anesthetics and Other Medications.")

Prolonged Seizures

Most ECT seizures are self-limited, lasting less than 2 minutes. In rare instances, however, persistent seizure activity (prolonged seizures and status

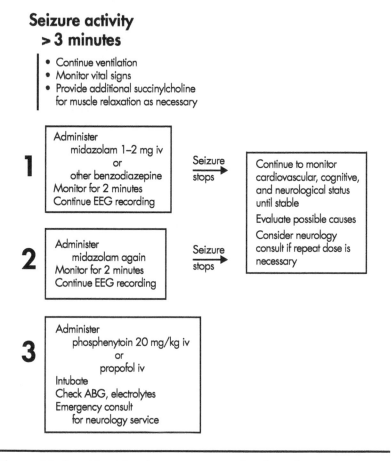

Figure 11–2.   Algorithm for management of prolonged seizures.

ABG=arterial blood gas; EEG=electroencephalogram; iv=intravenously.

epilepticus) or a recurrence of seizure activity (tardive seizures) may occur (Weiner et al. 1991). A prolonged seizure can be defined as seizure activity lasting longer than 3 minutes (American Psychiatric Association 2001). EEG monitoring is especially useful in detecting prolonged seizures, because most are undetectable by motor observation alone. Prolonged seizures are particularly likely to occur in one of the following circumstances: 1) at the first treatment,

2) during benzodiazepine withdrawal, 3) in patients in whom proconvulsant medications (e.g., caffeine, theophylline) and lithium are used concurrently, or 4) in patients who have epilepsy or preexisting paroxysmal EEG activity. Young patients, especially those with mania or schizophrenia, also appear to have a higher incidence of prolonged seizures.

Prolonged seizures should be terminated pharmacologically after 3 minutes of sustained seizure activity. Seizures can be terminated by intravenously administering either a repeat dose of the anesthetic agent (e.g., methohexital) or a short-acting benzodiazepine (e.g., 1–2 mg midazolam). If after 2 more minutes the seizure still has not aborted, the dose should be repeated. If the patient continues to experience seizure activity, immediate neurology consultation should be obtained, blood gases and electrolytes should be checked, and lorazepam (2–4 mg iv over 1 minute) or diazepam (5–10 mg iv) should be given. An algorithm for termination of prolonged seizures is provided in Figure 11–2. It is important that the patient continue to receive adequate oxygenation during a prolonged seizure; this may be accomplished via positive-pressure ventilation or by the placement of an endotracheal tube if either 1) the seizure activity is grossly prolonged (more than 5–10 minutes) or 2) the patient becomes significantly hypoxic. Adequate muscular relaxation should be ensured as well. Vital signs (particularly blood pressure, oxygen saturation, and electrocardiogram) should be monitored continuously. After the patient is stabilized, the cause of the prolonged seizure should be investigated. In most cases, ECT can safely be resumed, although concurrent use of an anticonvulsant agent may be indicated in some cases.

References

American Psychiatric Association: The Practice of Electroconvulsive Therapy: Recommendations for Treatment, Training, and Privileging (A Task Force Report of the American Psychiatric Association), 2nd Edition. Washington, DC, American Psychiatric Publishing, 2001

Bergsholm P, Gran L, Bleie H: Seizure duration in unilateral electroconvulsive therapy: the effect of hypocapnia induced by hyperventilation and the effect of ventilation with oxygen. Acta Psychiatr Scand 69:121–128, 1984

Brewer CL, Davidson JR, Hereward S: Ketamine ("Ketalar"): a safer anaesthetic for ECT. Br J Psychiatry 120:679–680, 1972

Calev A, Fink M, Petrides G, et al: Caffeine pretreatment enhances clinical efficacy and reduces cognitive effects of electroconvulsive therapy. Convuls Ther 9:95–100, 1993

Coffey CE, Figiel GS, Weiner RD, et al: Caffeine augmentation of ECT. Am J Psychiatry 147:579–585, 1990

Krystal AD, Weiner RD: ECT seizure therapeutic adequacy. Convuls Ther 10:153–164, 1994

Krystal AD, Weiner RD: ECT seizure duration: reliability of manual and computer automated determinations. Convuls Ther 11:158–169, 1995

Krystal AD, Coffey CE, Weiner, RD, et al: Changes in seizure threshold over the course of electroconvulsive therapy affect therapeutic response and are detected by ictal EEG ratings. J Neuropsychiatry Clin Neurosci 10:178–186, 1998

Krystal AD, Dean MD, Weiner RD, et al: ECT stimulus intensity: are present ECT devices too limited? Am J Psychiatry 157:963–967, 2000

Krystal AD, Weiner RD, Dean MD, et al: Comparison of seizure duration, ictal EEG, and cognitive effects with ketamine and methohexital anesthesia with ECT. J Neuropsychiatry Clin Neurosci 15:27–34, 2003

McCall WV, Reid S, Rosenquist P, et al: A reappraisal of the role of caffeine in ECT. Am J Psychiatry 150:1543–1545, 1993

Robin A, Binnie CD, Copas JB: Electrophysiological and hormonal responses to three types of electroconvulsive therapy. Br J Psychiatry 147:707–712, 1985

Sackeim HA, Decina P, Kanzler M, et al: Effects of electrode placement on the efficacy of titrated, low-dose ECT. Am J Psychiatry 144:1449–1455, 1987

Sackeim HA, Prudic J, Devanand DP, et al: Effects of stimulus intensity and electrode placement on the efficacy and cognitive effects of electroconvulsive therapy. N Engl J Med 328:839–846, 1993

Weiner RD, Coffey CE, Krystal AD: The monitoring and management of electrically induced seizures. Psychiatr Clin North Am 14:845–869, 1991

12

Index ECT

Mehul V. Mankad, M.D.

In addition to making the decisions discussed in previous chapters, the practitioner must also make a determination of how frequently the seizures should be induced (i.e., the interval between treatments) and how many treatments should be administered in the treatment course.

Frequency of Treatments

The optimal frequency of ECT has not yet been determined (Shapira et al. 1991). In the United States, most ECT treatments are given three times a week (e.g., Monday, Wednesday, and Friday), whereas in some other countries (e.g., the United Kingdom), they may be administered twice weekly. Although an increased frequency is associated with a more rapid response, it may also be associated with increased cognitive side effects (Lerer et al. 1995).

A three-times-weekly schedule appears to be an acceptable compromise for most patients. The practitioner should consider decreasing the treatment frequency to twice, or even once, weekly if cognitive side effects are severe. Alternatively, treatment frequency may be increased to daily if a more rapid response is urgently needed, particularly at a time early in the course of treatments.

Multiple Monitored ECT

Multiple monitored ECT (MMECT) was developed in an attempt to decrease the total duration of the treatment course by inducing multiple seizures (usually 2–10) during a single treatment (Blachly and Gowing 1966; Maletzky 1981; Roemer et al. 1990). MMECT has been associated with a more rapid clinical response (fewer treatment sessions), but the total number of seizures required is greater. Some evidence suggests that prolonged seizure activity, exaggerated cardiovascular responses, and increased cognitive side effects may occur more frequently with MMECT, at least when relatively large numbers of seizures are administered in a single session (Abrams 2002).

Number of Treatments

No set number of treatments is required to complete a full course of ECT. As soon as the patient is judged to have achieved a maximum clinical response, the ECT course is terminated. To determine that a maximum response has been attained, the practitioner needs to observe a plateau in the patient's improvement such that no additional benefit is apparent despite two or three additional treatments. Some practitioners find it useful to serially administer objective symptom scales, such as the Hamilton Rating Scale for Depression (Hamilton 1960) or the Montgomery-Åsberg Depression Rating Scale (Montgomery and Åsberg 1979), and/or global scales, such as the Clinical Global Impression (Overall and Gorham 1962), to assist in this process. A typical ECT course involves 6–12 treatments, although the number required may occasionally be as low as 3 or as high as 20.

For nonresponders, or patients whose clinical progress is minimal after approximately six treatments, alterations in the ECT course should be considered. Possible modifications include changing from unilateral to bilateral electrode placement, increasing stimulus intensity, or potentiating the seizure pharmacologically. If the patient still does not respond after three to four additional treatments, or if response has reached a plateau below a full level of remission by that point, the ECT course should be terminated.

References

Abrams R: Electroconvulsive Therapy, 4th Edition. New York, Oxford University Press, 2002

Blachly PH, Gowing D: Multiple monitored electroconvulsive treatment. Compr Psychiatry 7:100–109, 1966

Hamilton M: A rating scale for depression. J Neurol Neurosurg Psychiatry 23:56–62, 1960

Lerer B, Shapira B, Calev A, et al: Antidepressant and cognitive effects of twice- versus three-times-weekly ECT. Am J Psychiatry 152:564–570, 1995

Maletzky BM: Multiple-Monitored Electroconvulsive Therapy. Boca Raton, FL, CRC Press, 1981

Montgomery SA, Asberg M: A new depression scale designed to be sensitive to change. Br J Psychiatry 141:45–49, 1979

Overall JE, Gorham DR: The Brief Psychiatric Rating Scale. Psychol Rep 10:799–812, 1962

Roemer RA, Dubin WR, Jaffe R, et al: An efficacy study of single- versus double-seizure induction with ECT in major depression. J Clin Psychiatry 51:473–478, 1990

Shapira B, Calev A, Lerer B: Optimal use of electroconvulsive therapy: choosing a treatment schedule. Psychiatr Clin North Am 14:935–946, 1991

13

Maintenance ECT

Mehul V. Mankad, M.D.

Most psychiatrists agree that following the remission of a depressive episode, therapy should be continued for at least 6–12 months. After the conclusion of a course of ECT, three options are available for continued treatment: administration of applicable psychotropic medications (e.g., antidepressant, antimanic, and/or antipsychotic agent), administration of continuation ECT, and psychotherapy combined with either medication or continuation ECT. A fourth option, involving the use of both continuation medication and ECT, may be necessary for patients with a history of failure of prophylaxis with either treatment alone.

Multiple psychiatric disorders, including major depressive disorder, psychotic depression, bipolar disorder, and schizoaffective disorder, respond to maintenance ECT (Birkenhager et al. 2005). Use of maintenance ECT in the geriatric population is also well documented (Thienhaus et al. 1990). Particular forms of schizophrenia (catatonia, refractory positive symptoms) may also be responsive to the combination of ECT and antipsychotic medication (Shimizu et al. 2007; Suzuki et al. 2006) (see Chapter 2, "Indications for Use").

Pharmacotherapy Without Maintenance ECT

Several studies have found that patients who were initially drug refractory have a higher risk of relapse within the first 12 months than do those who received ECT on a first-line basis, even with the posttreatment use of prophylactic pharmacotherapy (Sackeim et al. 1990, 1994). The drug-refractory patient should be placed on a different type of antidepressant from that used during the index episode, and/or continuation ECT should be considered.

Continuation ECT

Many practitioners have found an improvement of relapse rates when continuation ECT is performed (Monroe 1991). As summarized in Table 13–1, criteria for continuation ECT should include all of the following: a history of recurrent illness that is acutely responsive to ECT; limited medical comorbidities that increase risk for additional ECT or anesthesia; ineffectiveness or intolerance to prophylaxis with pharmacotherapy (or patient preference for ECT); and ability and willingness to comply with logistical arrangements (because continuation treatments are almost always performed on an outpatient basis) (American Psychiatric Association 2001; Fink et al. 1996).

Although an optimal protocol for timing of treatments still remains to be determined, a typical arrangement would involve weekly ECT for 4 weeks, then incremental increases in the interval between ECT treatments to once a month over the next few months (Clarke et al. 1989). Also, regardless of the system used routinely, flexibility in the choice of intertreatment intervals is necessary, given fluctuation in the patient's clinical status. If a significant and sustained increase in symptoms suggests a relapse or impending relapse, the practitioner should consider an increase in the frequency of treatments.

Maintenance ECT

Because a strict delineation between continuation ECT and maintenance ECT does not exist, some ECT programs do not recognize a distinction between the two. Due to the severity and chronicity of some patients' illnesses, many practitioners continue ECT for longer periods, particularly when attempts to discontinue therapy have resulted in a recurrence of the illness.

Table 13–1. Criteria for continuation ECT

- Positive response to index ECT for a recurrent psychiatric illness
- Limited medical comorbidities that increase risk for additional ECT or anesthesia
- Failure of pharmacotherapy (or patient preference for additional ECT)
- Ability and willingness to comply with logistical arrangements for outpatient ECT

The frequency of maintenance treatments should be determined based on the history of the patient's response to maintenance ECT, the patient's current level of severity, the degree of cognitive impairment, and practical considerations (e.g., availability of transportation). For patients in whom relapse reliably occurs when the interval between treatments exceeds a particular period of time, the treatment intervals should be based on this information. As with continuation ECT treatments, a significant and sustained increase in severity should trigger an increase in the frequency of maintenance treatments. In some patients, however, the degree of cognitive side effects can limit how frequently ECT can be administered.

Taking the above-mentioned factors into account, the average interval between maintenance ECT treatments is roughly 1 month, although the range is substantial. Given the increased interval between ECT treatments, the intrinsic anticonvulsant effect of ECT may wane. Some ECT programs advocate retitration of the seizure threshold during the maintenance phase (Wild et al. 2004).

There is no lifetime maximum number of ECT treatments for patients (Russell et al. 2003; Wijkstra and Nolen 2005). Cumulative amnestic effects do not appear likely except when the frequency of treatments remains high, although cognitive recovery from the index course may be slowed (Abraham et al. 2006; Datto et al. 2001; Rami et al. 2004).

Preanesthesia Reevaluation

Determination and documentation of the continued need for treatment should be made periodically on the basis of an assessment of relevant benefits and risks, and informed consent should be reobtained at least every 6 months (American Psychiatric Association 2001). A brief review of the patient's medical and mental status during the past interval should be done before each treatment. The risks and benefits of maintenance therapy should be evaluated on an ongoing basis. Routine laboratory data for ECT are usually updated at least yearly. Some programs choose to formalize this process and repeat preoperative screening at a specific interval. If significant events in the patient's medical history arise between maintenance treatments (e.g., myocardial infarction, new-onset diabetes mellitus), then reassessment of those issues must be addressed prior to the next scheduled treatment.

References

Abraham G, Milev R, Delva N, et al: Clinical outcome and memory function with maintenance electroconvulsive therapy: a retrospective study. J ECT 22:43–45, 2006

American Psychiatric Association: The Practice of Electroconvulsive Therapy: Recommendations for Treatment, Training, and Privileging (A Task Force Report of the American Psychiatric Association), 2nd Edition. Washington, DC, American Psychiatric Publishing, 2001

Birkenhager TK, van den Broek WW, Mulder PG, et al: One-year outcome of psychotic depression after successful electroconvulsive therapy. J ECT 21:221–226, 2005

Clarke TB, Coffey CE, Hoffman GW, et al: Continuation therapy for depression using outpatient electroconvulsive therapy. Convuls Ther 5:330–337, 1989

Datto CJ, Levy S, Miller DS, et al: Impact of maintenance ECT on concentration and memory. J ECT 17:170–174, 2001

Fink M, Abrams R, Bailine S, et al: Ambulatory electroconvulsive therapy: report of a task force of the Association for Convulsive Therapy. Convuls Ther 12:42–55, 1996

Monroe RR Jr: Maintenance electroconvulsive therapy. Psychiatr Clin North Am 14:947–960, 1991

Rami L, Bernardo M, Boget T, et al: Cognitive status of psychiatric patients under maintenance electroconvulsive therapy: a one-year longitudinal study. J Neuropsychiatry Clin Neurosci 16:465–471, 2004

Russell JC, Rasmussen KG, O'Connor MK, et al: Long-term maintenance ECT: a retrospective review of efficacy and cognitive outcome. J ECT 19:4–9, 2003

Sackeim HA, Prudic J, Devanand DP, et al: The impact of medication resistance and continuation pharmacotherapy on relapse following response to electroconvulsive therapy in major depression. J Clin Psychopharmacol 10:96–104, 1990

Sackeim HA, Long J, Luber B, et al: Physical properties and quantification of the ECT stimulus, I: basic principles. Convuls Ther 10:93–123, 1994

Shimizu E, Imai M, Fujisaki M, et al: Maintenance electroconvulsive therapy (ECT) for treatment-resistant disorganized schizophrenia. Prog Neuropsychopharmacol Biol Psychiatry 31:571–573, 2007

Suzuki K, Awata S, Takano T, et al: Adjusting the frequency of continuation and maintenance electroconvulsive therapy to prevent relapse of catatonic schizophrenia in middle-aged and elderly patients who are relapse-prone. Psychiatry Clin Neurosci 60:486–492, 2006

Thienhaus OJ, Margletta S, Bennett JA: A study of the clinical efficacy of maintenance ECT. J Clin Psychiatry 51:485–486, 1990

Wijkstra J, Nolen WA: Successful maintenance electroconvulsive therapy for more than seven years. J ECT 21:171–173, 2005

Wild B, Eschweiler GW, Bartels M: Electroconvulsive therapy dosage in continuation/ maintenance electroconvulsive therapy: when is a new threshold titration necessary? J ECT 20:200–203, 2004

14

Step-by-Step Outline of ECT Administration

The following outline serves as a comprehensive overview of a typical ECT treatment procedure, summarizing many of the recommendations made elsewhere in this volume. The goal is not to create a standard of practice but rather to provide the practitioner with an overall perspective about the treatment procedure. Many of these recommendations must be adapted to the specific treatment site and the individual needs of each patient.

Part 1: Pre-ECT Evaluation

Evaluation for ECT can take place in an inpatient or an outpatient setting. Because length-of-stay considerations are becoming more important in the present era of health care reform, preparation of inpatients for ECT should be carried out promptly, in some cases even before hospitalization. Preauthorization of ECT has become essential for reimbursement from third-party payers.

Table 14–1. Major components of pre-ECT evaluation

1. Delineate indications for treatment: perform psychiatric history and exam.
2. Delineate risks: perform medical history and exam with laboratory evaluation.
3. Order any other medical consultations that may be indicated.
4. Perform risk-benefit analysis.
5. Perform patient (and, if applicable, family) education as part of informed consent procedure.
6. Determine whether ECT should be administered and, if so, whether it should be initiated on an inpatient or outpatient basis.
7. Recommend type of ECT (bilateral or unilateral) and any modifications in the ECT procedure.
8. Recommend any indicated modification(s) in the patient's medication or treatment regimen before ECT, including medications to be given on the day of treatment.
9. Document results of steps 1–8 in the medical record.

Major components of the pre-ECT evaluation (see Chapter 2, "Indications for Use," and Chapter 3, "Patient Referral and Evaluation") are listed in Table 14–1. Many of these components are typically written as orders to be done by persons other than the attending physician and the primary nurse(s) taking care of the patient. Sample orders of this type are provided in Table 14–2.

Table 14–2. Sample routine orders for pre-ECT evaluation

Essential orders

1. ECT consult (or second opinion): contact Dr. _____ (This may not be required, check hospital protocol and state laws.)
2. Consult anesthesiology for preoperative evaluation
3. Labs: complete blood count, serum electrolytes, other: _____
4. Electrocardiogram (if patient is older than 40 years)
5. Chest X ray (if patient has cardiovascular or pulmonary disease or a history of smoking)

Additional routine orders used by some practitioners

1. Routine electroencephalography
2. Memory or neuropsychological testing
3. Patient and family education (video, pamphlet, book, nursing teaching, etc.)

Before the first treatment, the following should be completed and documented:

- ECT consult (or second opinion, if applicable)
- Physical examination
- Anesthesia evaluation
- Patient education
- Informed consent
- Appropriate laboratory tests
- If indicated, other consultations

Some practitioners have found that a standardized pre-ECT evaluation summary sheet is useful.

Part 2: Patient Preparation on Day of Treatment

Preparation of inpatients on the day of treatment takes place on the ward. For outpatients, this preparation begins at home and continues in a designated pre-ECT area such as a freestanding ECT suite, a partial hospital unit, an inpatient ward, or a perioperative observation area. The following list of the components of this preparation is summarized in Table 14–3.

1. *Pre-ECT orders.* Pre-ECT orders should include the date and time of the first 1–3 treatments, requirements concerning oral intake before ECT, any medications required before entry into the treatment area or following return from that site, and instructions for vital signs and placement of the intravenous (iv) drip. Examples of basic pre-ECT orders are shown in Table 14–4 (inpatients) and Table 14–5 (outpatients).

Table 14–3.   Patient preparation on day of treatment

1.   Ensure that pre-ECT orders have been written (see Tables 14–4 and 14–5).
2.   Administer pre-ECT medications.
3.   Make sure bodily functions are attended to (urination, bowel movements).
4.   Ensure proper patient attire.
5.   Perform pre-ECT intake and interval assessment.

Table 14–4. Sample pre-ECT orders for inpatient

1. Schedule ECT for _____ (date or dates).
2. Allow nothing by mouth after midnight prior to treatment, except _____ medication to be given at _____ o'clock with a sip of water.
3. Insert saline lock iv before first treatment and maintain per protocol.
4. Assess vital signs, adverse effects, and orientation status pre- and post-ECT per protocol.
5. Administer glycopyrrolate 0.2 mg intramuscularly 30 minutes before ECT (if intramuscular anticholinergic premedication is used).
6. Give _____ medications on return from ECT (if indicated).

2. *Administration of pre-ECT medications.* Medications given by mouth, whether at home or in the hospital, should be taken with only a sip of water.
3. *Attention to bodily functions.* Care must be taken to ensure not only that patients have not taken anything by mouth the morning of ECT, but also that they have voided within a couple of hours of the procedure.
4. *Patient attire.* Before entry into the treatment room, patients in most facilities are asked to dress in a hospital gown, although some facilities allow loose-fitting street clothes. All jewelry (including facial piercing jewelry), makeup, dentures, dental appliances, and hearing aids should be removed. The patient's hair should be dry and free of exogenous substances (washing the hair on the night before ECT is helpful). If jewelry cannot be removed (e.g., tight wedding band), it should be covered with tape so that no bare metal is visible.

Table 14–5. Sample pre-ECT orders for outpatient

1. Schedule ECT for _____ (date or dates).
2. Admit to ECT service on day of treatment per protocol.
3. Allow nothing by mouth after midnight prior to treatment, except _____ medication to be given at _____ o'clock with a sip of water.
4. Insert saline lock iv before each treatment and maintain per protocol.
5. Assess vital signs, adverse effects, and orientation status pre- and post-ECT per protocol.
6. Administer glycopyrrolate 0.2 mg intramuscularly 30 minutes before ECT (if intramuscular anticholinergic premedication is used).
7. Give _____ medications on return from ECT (if indicated).
8. Discharge patient from ECT service when routine discharge criteria are met.

5. *Pre-ECT intake and interval assessment.* For patients who will be receiving their first treatment, the results of the pre-ECT evaluation should be checked. Regardless of the treatment number, an assessment (before entry into the ECT treatment area) should be done to determine that the patient is indeed prepared for the ECT treatment on that day and that no new developments preclude its administration. This assessment should include verification that all components included in steps 1–4 above have been satisfactorily completed, plus a brief direct patient evaluation. For inpatients, this task is generally accomplished on the ward and is documented either in a progress note or on a standardized pre-ECT checklist that can be performed by the nursing staff. For outpatients, this assessment is completed by nursing or medical staff in the pre-ECT staging area. Because outpatients have generally been away from direct medical observation for 2 or more days between treatments, they should also be given a brief interval psychiatric and medical examination including vital signs and baseline mental status (orientation). This examination should focus on areas of importance to both therapeutic outcome and treatment risk.

Part 3: Patient Preparation in Treatment Room

The following is a list of suggestions for preparation of the patient in the treatment area. Table 14–6 provides a summary of these recommendations.

1. *Ascertain that items 1–5 in the previous section, "Part 2: Patient Preparation on Day of Treatment," have been satisfactorily completed and documented.*
2. *Be aware of and respond to the patient's feelings and concerns.* In addition to the specific steps involved in this preparation process, pay attention to the manner in which the treatment team relates to the patient during this period, which is often marked by a considerable degree of anxiety, particularly at the first treatment. The staff should focus on the patient's specific physical, emotional, and educational needs, as well as on the technical requirements of the ECT preparation process. The staff should discuss what they are doing with the patient in easily understood terms (e.g., referring to "heart wave" and "brain wave" recording electrodes) and should answer any questions about the procedure. Because amnesia may develop during ECT, the staff should repeat such material to the patient during

subsequent treatments. If a patient is extremely anxious, the staff may need to delay placement of electroencephalographic (EEG) and stimulus electrodes until the patient is asleep.

3. *Position the patient on a bed or stretcher.* Patients may walk to the treatment room unless they have a physical handicap that would prevent them from doing so; however, many hospitals prefer that patients be transported by wheelchair, as they would be for many other procedures or tests. The treatment bed or stretcher should be capable of elevating the patient's head or feet and should also be electrically insulated to prevent the possibility of the current being grounded through the patient.

4. *Examine the patient's mouth.* Check to make sure that dentures or other dental appliances have been removed, and note any chipped or loose teeth or other significant problems within the oral cavity. In some cases, dental or oral abnormalities may require changes in the type of mouthpiece used (see "Part 4: Treatment," below).

5. *Check vital signs.* As discussed in Chapter 9, "Cardiovascular Response," heart rate and blood pressure vary considerably during the treatment. The anesthesiologist usually keeps a record of the patient's vital signs and reactions at different times during the procedure, although this responsibility is sometimes assigned to another staff member. Vital signs are measured serially over the time the patient is in the treatment area. One typical protocol involves measurements at several times:
   - On arrival in the treatment room
   - Just before stimulation
   - 30 seconds and 1, 3, and 5 minutes after stimulation
   - Just before leaving the treatment room
   Remember: The blood pressure cuff used for monitoring should not be placed on the arm with the intravenous (iv) drip or the oximetry sensor.

6. *Insert an iv catheter into an accessible vein in the hand or arm (unless already done).* This iv site should be maintained until the patient has returned to baseline pulmonary and cardiovascular status.

7. *Apply electrocardiographic (ECG) electrodes and check baseline recording for rate and rhythm.* These electrodes are usually placed over the right shoulder, the left shoulder, and the apex of the heart. Monitoring is carried out using ECG recording circuitry built into the ECT device or external equipment.

8. *Apply pulse oximetry sensor.* The oximetry sensor, generally in the form of a clip attachment, should be positioned on a fingertip. The patient's baseline oxygen saturation should be obtained. Serial monitoring should be obtained at the same intervals as vital signs while the patient is in the treatment area.

9. *Apply EEG electrodes.* For EEG monitoring, disposable pediatric ECG electrodes are often used because of their small size and ease of attachment. For two-channel EEG monitoring, the four electrodes should be placed on a cleansed skin surface (see Chapter 8, "Ictal Electroencephalographic Response") with their midpoints 1 inch above the midpoint of each eyebrow and behind both ears on the rostral portion of the mastoid process (see Figure 8–3 in Chapter 8). Care should be taken to ensure that the tips of the electrode leads are plugged into the monitoring cable so that the left- and right-side recording electrodes are each connected to a separate recording channel on the output display of the ECT device. To keep track of which channel is left and which is right, both electrodes and the receptive ends of the monitoring cables should be labeled. Tapping each electrode sequentially and observing the EEG chart recorder/monitor display to see where the tap artifact shows up is also useful.

   If one-channel EEG monitoring is performed, electrodes should be placed in the left prefrontal area and behind the left ear (mastoid process). This placement helps to ensure that a generalized bilateral seizure has occurred with right unilateral ECT.

10. *Apply electromyographic (EMG) leads or optical motion sensor (if used).* When used, EMG leads are typically placed approximately 3 or more inches apart, distal to the blood pressure cuff that will be used for the cuff technique (described in Chapter 7 "Ictal Motor Response," and noted briefly below in "Part 4: Treatment"). At least one of the EMG electrodes should be placed directly over muscle tissue (see Figure 7–1 in Chapter 7). The optical motion sensor, if used, should be secured to a digit distal to the cuff.

11. *Prepare the leg for the cuff technique.* Apply a blood pressure cuff to one ankle. If the patient is receiving unilateral ECT, place the cuff on the lower extremity ipsilateral to the electrode placement (i.e., if the patient is receiving right unilateral ECT, place the cuff on the right ankle). Ipsilateral cuff placement will allow observation of the seizure in the contralateral hemisphere. This approach allows confirmation of seizure

activity in the hemisphere that is not being directly stimulated. To minimize discomfort to the patient, do not inflate the cuff until the treatment session is under way.

12. *Prepare the scalp and apply stimulus electrodes.* The skin over which stimulus electrodes will be placed is typically prepared while the patient is awake; however, the ECT practitioner has the option of waiting to apply the stimulus electrodes on the patient's scalp until the patient is sedated or fully anesthetized. Waiting to apply the stimulus electrodes may be helpful for particularly anxious patients.

Stimulus electrode placement for ECT can be divided into two categories: bilateral and nondominant unilateral (stimulation of the cerebral hemisphere opposite that involved in mediating language functions). The decision about which technique to use should be made during the pre-ECT evaluation (a more complete discussion of this topic can be found in Chapter 5, "Clinical Applications"). With bilateral ECT, both stimulus electrodes are typically attached by a headband. With unilateral ECT, only the frontotemporal electrode is placed in the headband and a handheld electrode is used for the homologous centroparietal position. Some practitioners choose to avoid use of the headband altogether and administer the ECT stimulus using two handheld electrodes. In such cases, the stimulus is generally activated by use of a remote treatment button located on one of the handheld electrodes or by use of a foot switch (alternatively, a second practitioner could initiate the stimulus by pushing the stimulus button on the ECT device itself). To minimize patient anxiety, application of the handheld electrodes is usually delayed until just before stimulation.

a. *Bilateral placement.* In bilateral electrode placement, the midpoints of the left and right stimulus electrodes are positioned approximately 1 inch (usually half the diameter of the electrode) above the middle of an imaginary line drawn between the upper tragus of the ear and the external canthus of the eye, as noted in Figure 14–1A.

b. *Unilateral placement.* In unilateral ECT, both stimulus electrodes are located over the nondominant hemisphere. (See Chapter 5 for a more complete discussion of the determination of hemispheric dominance.) A variety of unilateral positions can be used, but the d'Elia position

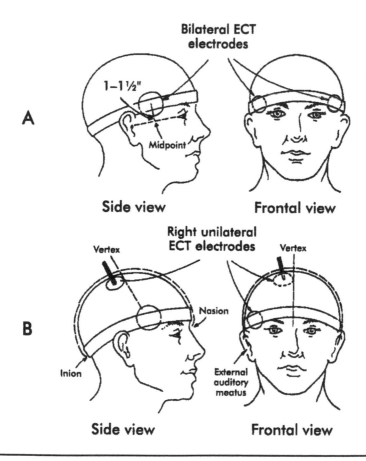

Figure 14–1. Electroconvulsive therapy electrode placement.

(A) Bilateral; (B) right unilateral.

is preferred (Figure 14–1B). This configuration involves placing one electrode over the presumed nondominant frontotemporal area, as in bilateral ECT. The other electrode is placed on the same side, centered 1 inch (typically half the diameter of the electrode) lateral to the vertex of the head. The vertex is defined as the intersection of the midpoints of two arcs: 1) the arc between the *inion* (the external occipital protuberance) and the *nasion* (the point where the bridge of the nose meets the skull) and 2) the arc between the two external auditory meati. In most cases, the electrodes end up being about 4–5 inches apart. Because interelectrode distance may be an important factor in treatment adequacy with unilateral ECT, it is important to measure the location of the vertex. A small dot made at the time of the first treatment with an indelible marker can minimize the need for repeated measurement.

After the placement sites for the stimulus electrodes have been determined, the skin underlying those sites should be cleaned. This may be done by rubbing the sites with alcohol, then allowing the area to dry. Many practitioners prefer a gritty skin cleanser (e.g., Omni Prep), which may improve electrical contact with the electrode. When this type of material is used, the skin should be wiped dry before electrodes are applied.

In general, steel discs are used as the stimulus electrodes, although the manufacturer Somatics (http://www.thymatron.com) also makes disposable adhesive pad electrodes for use with their devices. Two types of steel electrodes are used: flat, for placement in frontotemporal areas, and concave, for placement in the centroparietal location in unilateral ECT. Conductive gel is applied to each disc. The gel should be sufficient to completely cover the surface of the electrode but not exude excessively from around the edges when placed on the scalp.

The headband should be stretched snugly around the patient's head to prevent the electrodes from moving during treatment, but not so tightly that the patient is uncomfortable. It is important that the band be placed below the inion, the external occipital protuberance on the back of the head, so the band does not slip off when the neck is extended during the treatment.

In unilateral ECT, the centroparietal stimulus electrode site is also cleansed. Some practitioners spray on a fine saline solution to improve the electrical contact, taking care to avoid having the solution dampen an area larger than the actual contact zone, and/or rub a small amount of gel directly onto the contact area. Clipping or shaving the hair at the centroparietal site may be helpful if the hair is extremely thick, although most patients do not find this practice acceptable.

Table 14–6.   Patient preparation in treatment room

1. Ascertain that items 1–5 in "Part 2: Patient Preparation on Day of Treatment" in this chapter have been satisfactorily completed and documented.

2. Be aware of and respond to the patient's feelings and concerns.

3. Position the patient on a bed or stretcher.

4. Examine the patient's mouth.

5. Check vital signs.

6. Insert an intravenous catheter (unless already done in pre-ECT staging area).

7. Apply electrocardiographic electrodes and check baseline recording.

8. Apply pulse oximetry sensor.

9. Apply electroencephalographic electrodes.

10. Apply electromyographic leads or optical motion sensor, if either is used.

11. Prepare the leg for the cuff technique.

12. Prepare the scalp and apply stimulus electrodes.

13. Set stimulus parameters.

---

13. *Set stimulus parameters.* Stimulus parameters are set according to either a dose-titration paradigm or a fixed-dose paradigm. (See Chapter 5 for a review of stimulus dosing recommendations.)

Part 4: Treatment

An outline of the treatment protocol is discussed in this section and summarized in Table 14–7.

1. *Prior to administration of any medications, perform a "time-out" procedure.* The ECT team and the anesthesia team must be present during the time-out. The patient's name should be confirmed along with a secondary identifier, such as the date of birth or medical record number. The written informed consent should be located and verified. The location and type of procedure (i.e., electrode placement) should be confirmed. The anesthesia plan of care may be discussed as well. The time-out is also a good opportunity to briefly discuss with anesthesia colleagues any relevant issues from previous treatments that may have an impact on the current treatment (e.g., a suggested change in anesthetic to optimize seizure length).

Table 14–7.   Treatment protocol

1. Assemble the ECT team and anesthesia team for the "time-out" procedure, which involves confirming the name of the patient and a secondary identifier (medical record number, date of birth), type of procedure, and location of the procedure. The anesthesia plan of care may also be reviewed. Signed consent should be located and confirmed to be current.

2. Administer prophylactic medications.

3. Begin oxygenation.

4. Administer the anesthetic agent.

5. Observe the patient for action of the anesthetic agent.

6. Initiate the cuff technique.

7. Administer the muscle relaxant.

8. Observe the patient for action of the muscle relaxant.

9. Insert the bite block, and position the patient and the stimulus electrodes.

10. Test static impedance. (If using a machine with automatic impedance test, then confirm the value.)

11. Administer the stimulus.

12. Remove the bite block, quickly check the oral cavity, and resume oxygenation.

13. Evaluate the seizure response.

14. Deflate the cuff.

15. Verify the seizure completion.

16. Document the medications, stimulus parameters, seizure response, and vital signs.

17. Transfer the patient to the recovery area.

2. *Administer prophylactic medications.* If anticholinergic prophylaxis is desired, an iv or intramuscular (im) dose of glycopyrrolate (Robinul) or atropine can be given 30 minutes to 1 hour before the treatment. This pretreatment medication should be noted on the pre-ECT medical record. Anticholinergic medications are discussed in Chapter 6, "Anesthetics and Other Medications." Sympatholytic agents or other cardiac protective medications are also sometimes given intravenously before anesthesia induction to prophylactically control excessive hypertension or tachyarrhythmias during ECT (see Chapter 6). When such an agent is used, vital signs should be rechecked 2–3 minutes after administration to evaluate the patient's response before administration of the anesthetic agent.

3. *Begin oxygenation.* Oxygen is administered via a mask, starting before anesthesia induction. Some patients experience anxiety or claustrophobia when a mask is placed over the nose and mouth; therefore, the mask can be held a few inches away until these patients are anesthetized. Once the patient becomes apneic following the action of the anesthetic and muscle relaxant agents, ventilation is augmented by positive pressure, typically by bag-mask ventilation. For patients who will receive a nondepolarizing neuromuscular blocker such as cisatracurium (Nimbex), alternate airway management such as intubation may be considered. As noted earlier, pulse oximetry is used on all patients, via a finger clip sensor, to monitor oxygen saturation levels.

4. *Administer the anesthetic agent.* Methohexital (Brevital) (starting dose= 0.75–1.0 mg/kg of body weight) is the most commonly used anesthetic. (See Chapter 6 for alternative medications.) Some patients may complain of a burning or stinging sensation in the arm. This is a short-lived phenomenon produced by vascular irritation following the iv bolus and can often be prevented by dilution of the agent. The catheter should be flushed after the infusion. For benzodiazepine-dependent patients, flumazenil (Romazicon) may be administered intravenously after delivery of the primary anesthetic agent.

5. *Observe the patient for action of the anesthetic agent.* Indicators of the action of the anesthetic agent (not all of which will be present in all cases) include the following:
   - The patient becomes unresponsive to commands.
   - Yawning occurs.
   - Airway obstruction occurs, indicated by noisy, snoring respirations.
   - The eyelash reflex disappears.

6. *Initiate the cuff technique.* A blood pressure cuff placed on an extremity (ipsilateral to the stimulus electrodes with unilateral ECT) should be inflated to about 200 mm Hg after induction of anesthesia (see Chapter 7). This prevents the muscle relaxant from reaching muscles distal to the cuff, thus allowing the observation of the motor component of the seizure.

7. *Administer the muscle relaxant.* Succinylcholine (Anectine) (starting dose=0.5–1.25 mg/kg of body weight) is the most commonly used muscle relaxant (see Chapter 6). It should be administered in a rapid iv bolus.

Most anesthesiologists wait until an acceptable level of anesthesia has been obtained before administering the relaxant. Others administer the relaxant immediately following infusion of the anesthetic agent, particularly for patients in whom prior treatments have demonstrated that the anesthetic dosage is sufficient and that an adequate airway can be ensured. In either case, the iv catheter should be flushed again with saline following the infusion.

8. *Observe the patient for action of the muscle relaxant.* Succinylcholine (Anectine) causes depolarization of muscle fibers, termed fasciculations, in most patients (see Chapter 6). Fasciculations are fine twitching movements, initially noted on the head, neck, and upper extremities, which gradually progress to the lower extremities. Because some patients do not display prominent fasciculations, the following measures can also be used to assess adequate muscle relaxation:

  • The joints becoming freely movable from loss of muscle tone
  • The absence of a plantar withdrawal response
  • The disappearance of deep tendon reflexes

  A peripheral nerve stimulator applied over the posterior tibial nerve at the ankle or over the median or radial nerve at the wrist may also be used to monitor the level of muscular relaxation. When used, such stimulation should not be activated until the patient is anesthetized.

  A maximal state of relaxation occurs by the time fasciculations have disappeared (usually 1–3 minutes postinfusion), although adequate relaxation is often present shortly before this point. The window of time between achievement of adequate relaxation and regaining consciousness is often quite brief.

9. *Insert the bite block, and position the patient and the stimulus electrodes.* When adequate relaxation has been achieved, the ventilation is temporarily stopped and a rubber bite block or other protective device is carefully inserted between the teeth. Pressure is applied to the patient's jaw to bring the teeth into secure contact with the bite block, and the neck is extended. The tongue and gums should be clear of the teeth and bite block. If handheld electrodes are used, they are now placed in position. The individual managing the bite block and electrodes must be certain that his or her own hands are clear of the exposed portions of the stimulus electrodes.

10. *Test static impedance.* Most contemporary U.S. ECT machines automatically check static impedance. With some older machines, static impedance needs to be tested prior to delivery of the electrical stimulus. High impedance (usually more than 3,000 Ω) usually indicates a poor electrical connection between the machine and the patient (e.g., the stimulus cable is not attached to the electrodes, the scalp is not properly prepared, the electrodes are slipping over the hair). Low impedance (usually less than 250 Ω) usually indicates an anomalous impedance path between the stimulus electrodes (e.g., sweat, smeared gel or other exogenous conducting substance). In either case, problems with static impedance should be checked and corrected before stimulation.

11. *Administer the stimulus.* The stimulus should never be delivered until *all* of the following five criteria have been met (these criteria also hold for any restimulation):

    - The person in contact with the patient's head is ready.
    - The patient is adequately anesthetized.
    - The patient's muscles are adequately relaxed.
    - Stimulus and recording electrodes are properly positioned.
    - The bite block or other dental appliance has been properly placed.

    The physician administering the treatment should let everyone else in the room know when he or she is ready to stimulate. Barring electrical malfunction, the stimulus button must be depressed through the entire stimulus cycle with all contemporary U.S. ECT machines, because removal of positive pressure will abort the stimulus. Devices made by MECTA (http://www.mectacorp.com) and Somatics (http://www.thymatron.com) precede the stimulus with a brief (about 1-second) delay. In both companies' devices, the delay time and the duration of current flow are each associated with different audible signals

12. *Remove the bite block, quickly check the oral cavity, and resume oxygenation.* Oxygenation of the patient should be continued by positive-pressure ventilation following each stimulation. This should be continued until spontaneous respiratory muscle movements are strong enough to maintain an adequate tidal volume.

13. *Evaluate the seizure response* (see Chapter 7 and Chapter 8). A general evaluation for adequacy includes the following:

a. *Verify that seizure activity has occurred.* The patient should demonstrate tonic-clonic movements (primarily in the cuffed extremity) or an unequivocal ictal EEG response. The patient may demonstrate muscular contraction during the electrical stimulus. This should not be confused with seizure activity.

b. *If no seizure occurred, restimulate the patient within 20–30 seconds at an increased stimulus intensity, unless either the device malfunctioned or the stimulus was accidentally aborted.* In such situations, restimulation, this time at the same intensity, should be carried out after the problem is resolved. The bite block should be carefully replaced before any restimulation.

c. *Measure the length of the seizure.* Observation of the seizure has two components: the motor response and the ictal response. Timing begins at the conclusion of the electrical stimulus and lasts through the termination of the tonic-clonic movements (motor response) and the disappearance of ictal EEG activity (ictal response). Seizures shorter than 20–25 seconds by either the motor or the EEG criterion can be assumed to be inadequate unless evidence indicates that they are clearly suprathreshold (see Chapter 11, "Managing the ECT Seizure").

d. *If an inadequate seizure occurred, restimulate the patient at least at a 50% higher level.* Because of a brief refractory period, the practitioner should wait 30–60 seconds before restimulating. Potential causes of inadequate seizures should be investigated, and seizure augmentation should be considered, particularly if maximum stimulus intensity has been reached (see Chapter 11). Adequate relaxation and anesthesia should be maintained during restimulation attempts; achieving this may occasionally require small additional boluses of anesthetic or muscle relaxant.

14. *Deflate the cuff after the seizure activity ends or as required to prevent perfusion complications in the cuffed extremity.*

15. *Verify the seizure completion.* Seizure activity may continue after the motor response has terminated. EEG monitoring (either auditory or visual) is necessary to determine the seizure end point (see Chapter 8). However, termination may not be clear in 10%–15% of all seizures. If termination

has not clearly occurred, monitoring should be continued. Volitional movements, spontaneous respiration, and awakening indicate that seizure activity has ceased.

16. *Document the medications, stimulus parameters, seizure response, and vital signs.* This documentation should be sufficient to allow a reasonable reconstruction of the treatment and its outcome, and provide information about any changes in medications, stimulus parameters, or other treatment-related factors that may be indicated at future treatments. If the patient had difficulty in regaining spontaneous respirations, a decreased dose of succinylcholine and/or anesthetic should be considered for the next treatment. If excessive motor activity occurred during the seizure, the dose of succinylcholine should probably be increased during the next treatment. Note whether any teeth were damaged during the procedure. Cardiovascular complications, such as arrhythmias or unduly severe or prolonged hypertensive episodes, should be noted. Consultations with a specialist should be obtained for unusual or potentially dangerous complications.

17. *Transfer the patient to the recovery area as soon as all three of the following criteria are fulfilled:*
    - Spontaneous breathing has resumed.
    - Vital signs are moving toward stability.
    - No complications require acute intervention.

    However, the criteria for such transfer do not include full return to consciousness.

Part 5: Patient Care in Recovery Area

When the patient is transported to the recovery area, the following actions should be taken:

1. Continue to monitor the patient's vital signs and mental status (orientation) at least every 10–15 minutes while the patient is in the recovery area (generally 15–20 minutes).

2. Remove the iv catheter after determining that the patient is medically stable, unless the catheter is to remain for the next treatment. (This step usually applies only to behaviorally stable patients receiving an index course of ECT.)

3. *Document the patient's response.* This step includes documentation of the following:

- Vital signs
- Mental status
- Occurrence of adverse effects
- Behavior (including presence of postictal delirium)
- Medications administered in the recovery room (especially any sedating or antihypertensive agents whose effects may still be present)
- Any other information that should be relayed to the staff in the post-recovery area

4. *Release the patient to the postrecovery area once vital signs and behavior are stable, unless complications requiring immediate medical intervention are present.* In most facilities, a formal signout by the anesthesiologist is required before such release.

Part 6: Postrecovery Care

The final step of ECT administration is postrecovery care, which consists of the following steps:

1. Return the patient to the ward (inpatients) or the postrecovery area (outpatients). The area used for outpatients can be a designated freestanding area, a portion of the inpatient unit, a partial hospital unit, or a perioperative observation unit.
2. Monitor the patient's vital signs and mental status (orientation) upon arrival in the postrecovery area and at least hourly.
3. Administer postrecovery medications.
4. Provide food and drink to the patient.
5. Document the patient's response. This step includes documentation of vital signs, mental status, behavior (including presence of postictal delirium), and medications administered in the postrecovery area.
6. Allow the patient to resume ward activities. If hospitalized, the patient is able to resume ward activities as tolerated after physiological and behavioral stability has been achieved. However, patients who received antihypertensive agents at the time of ECT should be considered at risk of

falling and managed accordingly until the effects of such agents have ended.

7. Discharge the patient from the postrecovery area. An outpatient can be discharged to care of the family or significant other as soon as the patient is behaviorally and physiologically stable. Usually, a signout from nursing and/or medical staff is required, as well as the provision of a formal discharge including limitations on activities, a contact person if problems occur, and detailed instructions to prepare the patient for the next ECT treatment (if applicable). Activities upon arrival home or other location should be as tolerated. The patient should not drive or work on the day of a treatment.

Continuing Medical Education Activities

A wide variety of continuing medical education (CME) and training activities on ECT exist, including didactic seminars, workshops, courses, symposia, and practical training experiences. Regularly occurring ECT-related offerings can be found in conjunction with the annual meetings of both the American Psychiatric Association and the Association for Convulsive Therapy (held concurrently). Weeklong practical training experiences at the following locations also exist at the time of this writing:

Columbia Eastside Medical Center (Georgia)

Gary Figiel, M.D., Director
Columbia Eastside Medical Center
2160 Fountain Drive
Snellville, GA 30078
Telephone: (770) 982-2340
Fax: (770) 972-0805

Note: 3- to 5-day course offered by individual arrangement.

Columbia University/New York State Psychiatric Institute

Mitchell Nobler, M.D., Director
Department of Biological Psychiatry
New York State Psychiatric Institute
722 West 168th Street
New York, NY 10032
Telephone: (212) 543-5617
Fax: (212) 543-5854

Note: 5-day course offered approximately four times per year; 40 hours CME credits.

Duke University Medical Center

Physician Fellowship

Richard Weiner, M.D., Ph.D., Director
Box 3309
Duke University Medical Center
Durham, NC 27710
Telephone: (919) 681-8742
Fax: (919) 681-8744
E-mail: rweiner@duke.edu

Note: 5-day course offered 20 times yearly; 40 CME credits.

Nursing Fellowship

Grace Gunderson-Falcone, R.N., M.S.N., A/GNP
Box 3309
Duke University Medical Center
Durham, NC 27710
Telephone: (919) 684-3996
Fax: (919) 681-7343
E-mail: falco003@mc.duke.edu

Note: 5-day course for nurses offered by individual arrangement.

Long Island Jewish/Hillside Medical Center

Samuel Bailine, M.D., Charles Kellner, M.D., Max Fink, M.D.,
   G. Petrides, M.D.
Long Island Jewish/Hillside Medical Center
Glen Oaks, NY 11004
Telephone: (516) 465-2512
Fax: (516) 862-8604

Note: 5-day course offered approximately six times per year by individual
   arrangement; CME credit available.

University of Michigan

Daniel F. Maixner, M.D., Director; Anne Flanagan, R.N., Director of
   Half-Day Training for Nurses
UH-9C Box 0120
1500 East Medical Center Drive
Ann Arbor, MI 48109
Telephone: (734) 936-4960
Fax: (734) 936-9983

Note: Course available upon request; 1-week course for those beginning
   an ECT practice and 1-day course for current ECT practitioners

Western Psychiatric Institute and Clinic/
University of Pittsburgh Medical Center

Petronilla Vaulx-Smith, M.D., Ph.D., Director
Room 1070
Electroconvulsive Therapy Services
Western Psychiatric Institute and Clinic
3811 O'Hara Street
Pittsburgh, PA 15213
Telephone: (412) 246-5063
Fax: (412) 246-5065
Email: vaulx-smithpm@upmc.edu

Note: 5-day course offered quarterly; 40 CME credits

Educational Materials

Materials for Health Care Providers

Books

Abrams R: Electroconvulsive Therapy, 4th Edition. New York, Oxford University Press, 2002

American Psychiatric Association: The Practice of Electroconvulsive Therapy: Recommendations for Treatment, Training, and Privileging, 2nd Edition. Washington, DC, American Psychiatric Publishing, 2001

Ottoson J-O: Ethics in Electroconvulsive Therapy. New York, Routledge, 2004

Shorter E, Healy D: Shock Therapy: A History of Electroconvulsive Treatment in Mental Illness. Piscataway, NJ, Rutgers University Press, 2007

Journal

The Journal of ECT (previously *Convulsive Therapy*, published quarterly). New York, Lippincott Williams & Wilkins

Materials for Patients and Families

Books

Dukakis K, Tye L: Shock: The Healing Power of Electroconvulsive Therapy. New York, Avery, 2006

Fink M: Electroshock: Healing Mental Illness. New York, Oxford University Press, 2002

Fink M: Electroconvulsive Therapy: A Guide for Professionals and Their Patients. New York, Oxford University Press, 2008

Video

Dukakis K: Shock. Dallas, TX, AMS Pictures, 2007

Twelve individuals who underwent ECT discuss the treatment and their psychiatric disorders. The video is based on the 2006 book, listed above, by Dukakis and Tye.

Patient Information Sheet

What Is ECT?

ECT is a treatment for severe episodes of major depression, mania, and some types of schizophrenia. It involves the use of a brief, controlled electrical current to produce a seizure within the brain. This seizure activity is believed to bring about certain biochemical changes that may cause your symptoms to diminish or even to disappear. A series of seizure treatments, generally 6–12, given at a rate of 3 per week, is required to produce such a therapeutic effect, although sometimes a smaller or larger number may be necessary.

How Is ECT Administered?

ECT is usually administered three times per week, on Monday, Wednesday, and Friday mornings. You will not eat or drink after midnight the night before each treatment. Before the treatment, a small needle is placed in an arm vein so that later, at the time of the treatment, the medications used to put you to sleep and relax your muscles can be given through that needle. The treatment itself is given in a special ECT treatment suite, located not far from the ward. ECT is administered by a team of doctors who have had specialized training and experience in this type of treatment. You will be brought into the treatment room and asked to lie down on a comfortable stretcher, after which a blood pressure cuff will be placed on your arm and ankle. A number of electrodes will be placed on your scalp, chest, and finger so that brain waves (electroencephalogram), heart waves (electrocardiogram), and body oxygen levels can be monitored and so that the electrical stimulus can later be given after you are asleep. You will then be provided oxygen to breathe by mask, and any pre-ECT medications, if indicated, will be given, followed by the anesthetic medication itself, which will put you to sleep.

Within a minute after the injection of the anesthetic medication, you will be asleep, and the medication being used to relax your muscles will be given. Within 1–3 minutes, your muscles will be relaxed. A controlled electrical stimulus, lasting a fraction of a second to several seconds, will then be applied across the two stimulus electrodes, which will be placed either on both temples (bilateral ECT) or on the right temple and top of the head (unilateral ECT). As will be described later, unilateral ECT has less effect on memory than bilateral ECT. However, some doctors believe that it may not be as effective in some patients. The electrical stimulus will trigger a seizure within the brain, which typically lasts around a minute. The muscular response to the seizure is greatly reduced by the muscle relaxant drug given before the stimulation. Very little body movement occurs.

A few minutes after the seizure, when you are breathing well on your own, you will be moved to a nearby room, where you will wake within 5–10 minutes. Because of the anesthetic drug and the effects of having had the seizure, you will temporarily feel somewhat groggy. Usually within 15–25 minutes after leaving the treatment room, you will be returned to your room (if you are an inpatient), or you will go to another area of the treatment suite (if you are an outpatient), where you will wait until you are ready to leave the hospital (typically about an hour).

Is ECT Effective?

Although there have been many advances in the treatment of mental disorders in recent years, ECT remains the most effective, fastest, and/or safest treatment for some cases, particularly when alternative treatments, usually medications, are either ineffective or not safe. Your doctor will discuss with you why ECT is being recommended in your case and what alternative treatments may be available. ECT is most effective in major depression, where it has a strong beneficial effect in up to 80%–90% of patients, depending on the case. Still, there is no guarantee that ECT or, for that matter, any other treatment will be effective. In addition, although a series of ECT treatments (or an alternative treatment) may bring an episode of illness to an end, it will not in itself prevent another episode from occurring weeks, months, or years later. Therefore, you and your doctor will need to consider additional treatment to follow any ECT that you receive. Such treatment generally consists of medication, psychotherapy, or additional ECT (given to you as an outpatient at a much less frequent rate).

Is ECT Safe?

All treatments have risks and side effects, as does no treatment at all. Before ECT, you will undergo a medical, psychiatric, and laboratory evaluation to make sure that the treatments can be administered in the safest, most effective manner possible. Your medications may also be adjusted to minimize the risk and maximize the effectiveness of the treatments. For most patients, the side effects of ECT are relatively minor. The risk of death is very rare—about 1 per 10,000 patients for typical cases, but can be higher for individuals with some serious coexisting medical illnesses. Serious complications, which are also quite rare, include temporary or permanent heart abnormalities; reactions to the medication used at the times of the treatment; injuries to muscle, bones, or other parts of the body; and greatly prolonged seizures or seizures occurring after the treatment. More common side effects involve headache, muscle soreness, nausea, confusion, and memory difficulties. Headache, muscle soreness, and nausea are usually mild and can be prevented or at least diminished by medications.

Confusion and memory problems may build up over a course of ECT, but they diminish as soon as the treatments have stopped. Because mental disorders themselves often have harmful effects on memory function, however, in the long term, some patients successfully treated with ECT actually report an improvement in memory. When memory problems do occur, they vary considerably from patient to patient, but the problems are usually greater for patients having a larger numbers of treatments or for patients who have both sides of the head stimulated (bilateral ECT). Because of the possibility of memory loss, important life decisions should be postponed until any major negative effects of ECT on memory have worn off (usually within 1–2 weeks following completion of the treatment course).

ECT-related memory problems can be of two types: 1) a difficulty remembering new information and 2) a loss of some memories from the past, particularly the recent past (e.g., during and just before receiving ECT). The ability to learn and remember new information typically returns to one's usual level over a period of days to weeks after ECT. The ability to remember material from the past—that is, before ECT—likewise tends to return to normal over a similar period, except that some memories from the recent past, mainly days to months before the treatments, may be delayed in recovery or even permanently lost. Patient surveys have indicated that most patients receiving ECT are not greatly disturbed by memory effects and would have ECT again if physicians recommended it.

Other Information About ECT

Please feel free to ask your doctors or nursing staff any questions you have about ECT. Various types of information, including videotapes, are available concerning this treatment. You should understand that ECT is a treatment to which you (or your legal guardian, if applicable) must consent on a voluntary basis, and that consent for future treatments can be withdrawn at your (or your guardian's) request at any time.

Sample ECT Consent Forms

Electroconvulsive Therapy (ECT) Consent Form: Acute Phase

Name of Patient: _____

My doctor, _____, has recommended that I receive treatment with electroconvulsive therapy (ECT). This treatment, including the risks and benefits that I may experience, has been fully described to me. I give my consent to be treated with ECT.

Whether ECT or an alternative treatment, like medication or psychotherapy, is most appropriate for me depends on my prior experience with these treatments, the features of my illness, and other considerations. Why ECT has been recommended for me has been explained.

ECT involves a series of treatments that may be given on an inpatient or outpatient basis. To receive each treatment I will come to a specially equipped area in this facility. The treatments are usually given in the morning. Because the treatments involve general anesthesia, I will have had nothing to eat or drink for several hours before each treatment. Before the treatment, a small needle will be placed in my vein so that I can be given medications. An anesthetic medication will be injected that will quickly put me to sleep. I will then be given another medication that will relax my muscles. Because I will be asleep, I will not experience pain or discomfort or remember the procedure. Other medications may also be given depending on my needs.

To prepare for the treatment, monitoring sensors will be placed on my head and body. Blood pressure cuffs will be placed on an arm and leg. This monitoring involves no pain or discomfort. After I am asleep, a carefully controlled amount of electricity will be passed between two electrodes that have been placed on my head.

I may receive bilateral ECT or unilateral ECT. In bilateral ECT, one electrode is placed on the left side of the head, the other on the right side. In unilateral ECT, both electrodes are placed on the same side of the head, usually the right side. Right unilateral ECT (electrodes on the right side) is likely to produce less memory difficulty than bilateral ECT. However, for some patients bilateral ECT may be a more effective treatment. My doctor will carefully consider the choice of unilateral or bilateral ECT.

The electrical current produces a seizure in the brain. The amount of electricity used to produce the seizure will be adjusted to my individual needs, based on the judgment of the ECT physician. The medication used to relax my muscles will greatly soften the contractions in my body that would ordinarily accompany the seizure. I will be given oxygen to breathe. The seizure will last for approximately 1 minute. During the procedure, my heart, blood pressure, and brain waves will be monitored. Within a few minutes, the anesthetic medications will wear off and I will awaken. I will then be observed until it is time to leave the ECT area.

The number of treatments that I will receive cannot be known ahead of time. A typical course of ECT is 6 to 12 treatments, but some patients may need fewer and some may need more. Treatments are usually given three times a week, but the frequency of treatment may also vary depending on my needs. If I need more than _____ treatments, my written consent will be reobtained.

ECT is expected to improve my illness. However, I understand that I may recover completely, partially, or not at all. After ECT, my symptoms may return. How long I will remain well cannot be known ahead of time. To make the return of symptoms less likely after ECT, I will need additional treatment with medication, psychotherapy, and/or ECT. The treatment I will receive to prevent the return of symptoms will be discussed with me.

Like other medical treatments, ECT has risks and side effects. To reduce the risk of complications, I will receive a medical evaluation before starting ECT. The medications I have been taking may be adjusted. However, in spite of precautions, it is possible that I will experience a medical complication. As with any procedure using general anesthesia, there is a remote possibility of death from ECT. The risk of death from ECT is very low, about 1 in 10,000 patients. This rate may be higher in patients with severe medical conditions. ECT very rarely results in serious medical complications, such as heart attack, stroke, respiratory difficulty, or continuous seizure. More often, ECT results in irregularities in heart rate and rhythm. These irregularities are usually mild and short lasting but in rare instances can be life threatening. With modern ECT technique, dental complications are infrequent and bone fractures or dislocations are very rare.

If serious side effects occur, I understand that medical care and treatment will be instituted immediately and that facilities to handle emergencies are available. I understand, however, that neither the institution nor the treating physicians are required to provide long-term medical treatment. I shall be responsible for the cost of such treatment whether personally or through medical insurance or other medical coverage. I understand that no compensation will be paid for lost wages or other consequential damages.

The minor side effects that are frequent include headache, muscle soreness, and nausea. These side effects usually respond to simple treatment. When I awaken after each treatment, I may be confused. This confusion usually goes away within 1 hour. During the treatment course I may have new difficulties in attention and concentration and other aspects of thinking. These problems rapidly go away after completion of ECT.

I understand that memory loss is a common side effect of ECT. The memory loss with ECT has a characteristic pattern, including problems remembering past events and new information. The degree of memory problems is often related to the number and type of treatments given. A smaller number of treatments is likely to produce less memory difficulty than a larger number. Shortly following a treatment, the problems with memory are greatest. As time from treatment increases, memory improves.

I may experience difficulties remembering events that happened before and while I received ECT. The spottiness in my memory for past events may extend back to several months before I received ECT, and, less commonly, for longer periods of time, sometimes several years or more. Although many of these memories should return during the first few months following my ECT course, I may be left with some permanent gaps in memory.

For a short period following ECT, I may also experience difficulty in remembering new information. This difficulty in forming new memories should be temporary and typically disappears within several weeks following the ECT course.

The majority of patients state that the benefits of ECT outweigh the problems with memory. Furthermore, most patients report that their memory is actually improved after ECT. Nonetheless, a minority of patients report problems in memory that remain for months or even years. The reasons for these reported long-lasting impairments are not fully understood. As with any medical treatment, people who receive ECT differ considerably in the extent to which they experience side effects.

Because of the possible problems with confusion and memory, I should not make any important personal or business decisions during or immediately after the ECT course. During and shortly after the ECT course, and until discussed with my doctor, I should refrain from driving, transacting business, or other activities for which memory difficulties may be troublesome.

The conduct of ECT at this facility is under the direction of Dr. _____. I may contact him/her at _____ if I have further questions.

I am free to ask my doctor or members of the ECT treatment team questions about ECT at this time or at any time during or following the ECT course. My decision to agree to ECT is being made voluntarily, and I may withdraw my consent for further treatment at any time.

I have been given a copy of this consent form to keep.

_____   _____
Signature   Date

Person Obtaining Consent:

_____   _____
Name   Signature

Electroconvulsive Therapy (ECT) Consent Form: Continuation/Maintenance Treatment

Name of Patient: _____

My doctor, _____, has recommended that I receive continuation or maintenance treatment with electroconvulsive therapy (ECT). This treatment, including the risks and benefits that I may experience, has been fully described to me. I give my consent to be treated with this type of ECT.

I will receive ECT to prevent return of my illness. Whether ECT or an alternative treatment, like medication or psychotherapy, is most appropriate for me at this time depends on my prior experience with these treatments in preventing the return of symptoms, the features of my illness, and other considerations. Why continuation/maintenance ECT has been recommended for me has been explained.

Continuation/maintenance ECT involves a series of treatments, with each usually separated in time by 1 or more weeks. Continuation/maintenance ECT is usually given for a period of several months or longer. These treatments may be given on an inpatient or outpatient basis.

To receive each continuation/maintenance treatment I will come to a specially equipped area in this facility. The treatments are usually given in the morning. Because the treatments involve general anesthesia, I will have had nothing to eat or drink for several hours before each treatment. Before the treatment, a small needle will be placed in my vein so that I can be given medications. An anesthetic medication will be injected that will quickly put me to sleep. I will then be given another medication that will relax my muscles. Because I will be asleep, I will not experience pain or discomfort or remember the procedure. Other medications may also be given depending on my needs.

To prepare for the treatment, monitoring sensors will be placed on my head and body. Blood pressure cuffs will be placed on an arm and leg. This monitoring involves no pain or discomfort. After I am asleep, a carefully controlled amount of electricity will be passed between two electrodes that have been placed on my head.

I may receive bilateral ECT or unilateral ECT. In bilateral ECT, one electrode is placed on the left side of the head, the other on the right side. In unilateral ECT, both electrodes are placed on the same side of the head, usually the right side. Right unilateral ECT (electrodes on the right side) is likely to produce less memory difficulty than bilateral ECT. However, for some patients bilateral ECT may be a more effective treatment. My doctor will carefully consider the choice of unilateral or bilateral ECT.

The electrical current produces a seizure in the brain. The amount of electricity used to produce the seizure will be adjusted to my individual needs, based on the judgment of the ECT physician. The medication used to relax my muscles will greatly soften the contractions in my body that would ordinarily accompany the seizure. I will be given oxygen to breathe. The seizure will last for approximately 1 minute. During the procedure, my heart, blood pressure, and brain waves will be monitored. Within a few minutes, the anesthetic medications will wear off and I will awaken. I will then be observed until it is time to leave the ECT area.

The number of continuation/maintenance treatments that I will receive will depend on my clinical course. Continuation ECT is usually given for at least 6 months. If it is felt that continuation ECT is helpful and should be used for a longer period (maintenance ECT), I will be asked to consent to the procedure again.

ECT is expected to prevent the return of my psychiatric condition. Although for most patients ECT is effective in this way, I understand that this cannot be guaranteed. With continuation/maintenance ECT I may remain considerably improved or I may have a partial or complete return of psychiatric symptoms.

Like other medical treatments, ECT has risks and side effects. To reduce the risk of complications, I will receive a medical evaluation before starting ECT. The medications I have been taking may be adjusted. However, in spite of precautions, it is possible that I will experience a medical complication. As with any procedure using general anesthesia, there is a remote possibility of death from ECT. The risk of death from ECT is very low, about one in 10,000 patients. This rate may be higher in patients with severe medical conditions.

ECT very rarely results in serious medical complications, such as heart attack, stroke, respiratory difficulty, or continuous seizure. More often, ECT results in irregularities in heart rate and rhythm. These irregularities are usually mild and short lasting, but in rare instances can be life threatening. With modern ECT technique, dental complications are infrequent and bone fractures or dislocations are very rare.

If serious side effects occur, I understand that medical care and treatment will be instituted immediately and that facilities to handle emergencies are available. I understand, however, that neither the institution nor the treating physicians are required to provide long-term medical treatment. I shall be responsible for the cost of such treatment whether personally or through medical insurance or other medical coverage. I understand that no compensation will be paid for lost wages or other consequential damages.

The minor side effects that are frequent include headache, muscle soreness, and nausea. These side effects usually respond to simple treatment.

When I awaken after each treatment, I may be confused. This confusion usually goes away within 1 hour.

I understand that memory loss is a common side effect of ECT. The memory loss with ECT has a characteristic pattern, including problems remembering past events and new information. The degree of memory problems is often related to the number and type of treatments given. A smaller number of treatments is likely to produce less memory difficulty than a larger number. Shortly following a treatment, the problems with memory are greatest. As time from treatment increases, memory improves.

I may experience difficulties remembering events that happened before and while I received ECT. The spottiness in my memory for past events may extend back to several months before I received ECT, and, less commonly, for longer periods of time, sometimes several years or more. Although many of these memories should return during the first few months following continuation/maintenance ECT, I may be left with some permanent gaps in memory.

For a short period following each treatment, I may also experience difficulty in remembering new information. This difficulty in forming new memories should be temporary and will most likely disappear following completion of continuation/maintenance ECT.

The effects of continuation/maintenance ECT on memory are likely to be less pronounced than those during an acute ECT course. By spreading treatments out in time, with an interval of a week or more between treatments, there should be substantial recovery of memory between each treatment.

Because of the possible problems with confusion and memory, it is important that I not drive or make any important personal or business decisions the day that I receive a continuation/maintenance treatment. Limitations on my activities may be longer depending on the side effects I experience following each treatment and will be discussed with my doctor.

The conduct of ECT at this facility is under the direction of Dr. _____. I may contact him/her at _____ if I have further questions.

I am free to ask my doctor or members of the ECT treatment team questions about ECT at this time or at any time during or following the ECT course. My decision to agree to continuation/maintenance ECT is being made voluntarily, and I may withdraw my consent for future treatment at any time.

I have been given a copy of this consent form to keep.

_____
Signature   Date

Person Obtaining Consent:

_____   _____
Name   Signature

Index

*Page numbers printed in **boldface** type refer to tables or figures.*